NEEDLE WORK

WICK WELKER

Demodocus Publishing

Demodocus Publishing

Needle Work

By Wick Welker

Published by Demodocus Publishing LLC.

PO Box 7235

Rochester MN, 55903

ISBN: 978-1-7355374-2-9

Cover art by Damonza

Again, to Danny Allen.

FOREWORD

As a critical care anesthesiologist, I've helped care for many ill people. It is a complex world full of tragedy, hope, success and failures. In preparing to write this story, I drew from various and diverse experiences I've had during my work as a physician. Almost every medical emergency that happens in the following pages are derived from real life experiences.

However, there is nothing in this story that is meant to parallel real people or real patients. I feel it is important to emphasize that this story is not a memoir or autobiography in any way. It is a work of fiction written in a fictitious first person narrative which does not reflect my opinions on medicine, patient care, mental illness, addiction, marriage, or life in any way.

I was inspired to write this story because I've always been fascinated with how otherwise well-meaning people can become something different than they intended. I remember reading Macbeth in high school and thinking: *Did he have to become that monster? Was he always bad or was it one incre-*

mental bad decision after another that transformed an otherwise good person?

Taking it a step further—under the wrong circumstances, can anyone become a Macbeth? And if so, what safeguards should be in place to protect us from becoming our own tragic hero?

Thank you for exploring these concepts with me. I hope you enjoy the story.

Wick Welker

Needle Work

CHAPTER ONE

I've looked into the eyes of people at the exact moment they die.

There's nothing that special about it.

When I watched my first patient die—his fingertips gripping the bed sheets like it would inexplicably halt his demise—I waxed with naive, freshman philosophy: was his soul lingering in that ashen face? Or was he already disembodied, looking down with benevolence on his doctors thumping on his chest like idiots?

Even worse for my existential crisis was watching him as blood occasionally reached his brain during CPR. With just a few chest pumps, a trickle of blood lapped on the shores of his consciousness sending primal impulses down the spinal cord. In a fleeting moment of insanity, his body reanimated, dancing like a marionette—unwittingly fighting us while we tried to save him. Once the compressions stopped, his limbs collapsed like a felled tree, and his eyes glazed into empty orbs of glass.

Were people alive sometime in between the madness of getting a pulse back—some sort of spectrum of death? Did their souls slurp back into the body like a ghost being whipped away from the celestial light in the ceiling?

I don't ask these questions anymore.

Not only because they're stupid questions but mostly because they don't matter. Sometimes patients live; sometimes they die. But mostly they die. And there's nothing special about either case.

Not all die, of course. But if your belly is swelling to the size of a beach ball because your liver can't keep water where it's supposed to be, you're probably going to die soon. It might not be this week, but you're not hanging around much longer —doesn't matter how much I pound and shock your chest, you'll shuffle off.

And whose fault is it?

Is it the patient's fault because they drank too much? Is it the doctor's fault because they didn't act fast enough? Maybe it's the researcher's fault for not understanding the disease. These are also questions I don't ask anymore, not only because they're stupid, but mostly because they don't matter.

When a fourteen year old boy is slammed through the emergency department doors, breathing tube clogged with blood, do these questions help him? When I flip him on his side, inspecting the spinal cord for injury and discover his brain herniating out of the back of his skull like strings of spaghetti, does it help if I ask why? Fifteen years after watching my first patient die, I watched that child's eyes at the exact same moment of death.

There was nothing that special about it.

It was an event as unceremonious as blinking—except he never opened his eyes again.

I LIKE TO SAY NOW, after everything that had happened, that it was because I walked too close to the line of death. I didn't just walk there, I *worked* there—living and breathing death on a daily basis for fifteen years. I ate lunch with severed limbs and dissecting aortas—had coffee with fulminant bacterial meningitis. When death becomes so routine, the boundaries between who is doing good and who is doing evil don't just blur—the distinction is ablated.

Here's a rationalization of mine to tuck away for later: when there are two opposing forces—sun and moon, bacteria or antibiotic, healer or killer—they become partners unto an end. The cycle of day, the cycle of sickness, the cycle of life—whatever. Why does the day end? When will my dying grandma get better? Why was that person killed on the street? When you linger on these questions too long, say fifteen years, the questions boil away and you're left with only raw concepts:

Sunset. Death. Killer.

And that's when you stop asking stupid questions.

A doctor who tries to save a person after they've been riddled with bullets would be pointless without the killer behind those bullets. We become partners with the killer, throwing the living into sharp relief to the loss of life. So I lived close to that line, all those nights pumping on people's chests. The distinction between me and the disease became less and less significant until I felt like a partner with the cirrhotic liver or in some sort of silent agreement with the gangster with a handgun: *I will keep doing my part if you keep doing yours. Deal?* Tragedy makes my job essential.

After fifteen years, there are no more questions, only mantras that I repeat to myself—mantras to find solace like the bottom of a shot glass:

There is no day without night.

There is no health without disease.

There is no life without a killer.

I particularly like this last one.

Because it's about me.

MOST PEOPLE DON'T REALLY KNOW what anesthesiologists do. "Oh," they say "you're a gas man. I had anesthesia when I had my wisdom teeth pulled. That's what you do?"

No.

You don't need an anesthesiologist to get some teeth pulled. All you need for that is a tank of laughing gas, a syringe of novocaine, and a good lawyer in case you manage to screw it up.

You need an anesthesiologist when you've accidentally removed your face with a shotgun instead of aiming it at a place that would actually end your life. Putting a breathing tube in someone goes from difficult to near impossible when they no longer have a face. When the beep of your oxygen saturation begins to have the pitch of a bass guitar, you learn pretty quick what an anesthesiologist does.

You need an anesthesiologist when you get drunk and go boating in the frigid Puget Sound—In the middle of winter. At 2 a.m. During a storm.

Among the long line of people keeping you alive—the coastguard, the flight medics, the ER docs and dozens of nurses—you'll need a gasman or woman to thread a central line into your heart and infuse your body with some of the most powerful medications in the world. We coax your blood vessels to constrict, convince your brain to stop swelling and negotiate the terms and conditions of cardiac contractility.

When those things don't work, we also thump on your chest a little.

You'll want to have an anesthesiologist around when you have a brain tumor the size of a walnut, flicking on your brainstem. When a surgeon decides to relieve you of that tumor, I'll be there to paralyze your body into a statue of flesh and bone. That way, the surgeon won't accidentally nick a cranial nerve and have you wake up with an eye that doesn't work. I'll keep your blood pressure in a nice little sweet spot: low enough to prevent massive hemorrhage into your medulla but high enough so you don't knock out your brain's executive functions. I'll keep the carbon dioxide levels in your blood at a cool 32 mmHg, making your brain slack enough to operate on but not so much that your meninges pull away on blood vessels, bleeding into your brain.

If on a delightful afternoon you take a stroll down to your local drug dealer but get stabbed thirty eight times instead of the dime bag which you intended, an anesthesiologist can help out. As you exsanguinate half a liter a minute into your belly, I'll fill you with blood: packed red, platelets, plasma—whatever you think you may need as you circle around the drain. I'll analyze your blood components, making dutiful note of the specific deficits so that once you're all patched together by the surgeons, you don't later ooze with under coagulated blood and die in the intensive care unit.

We're the doctors in the shadows, behind the curtains, behind the surgeons. We're mixing up epinephrine and antibiotic powder, floating balloons into your heart, measuring the exact pressure of air that is in your lungs every time you take a breath. We thread catheters up your jugular, measuring an infinitesimally small dip in oxygen content to know if your brain decides to stroke out right on the OR table.

Sometimes we do all of this without ever meeting you.

One day you're sailing the high seas on your new catamaran and the next morning you wake up in the ICU. Whatever the hell it is that happened, I was there, silently analyzing the gases in your blood, ventilating your waterlogged lungs and pumping your flailing heart all while the surgical team head-bobbed to the stylings of John Fogerty and talked about their new Teslas.

So why do I spell this all out? Is it because I've been jaded—unrecognized for fifteen years about what an anesthesiologist does? Is this my much anticipated manifesto about all the poor, rich, anesthesiologists out there?

No.

To work in this field, you get over a patient not having the first clue about what you're about to do to their diseased, paralyzed and unconscious body. I've seen the glazed, disinterested faces of patients turn to utter glee when they see their hero surgeons show up five minutes before surgery. I learned long ago that people don't actually care what anesthesiologists do.

I tell you all this for context.

Context is a helpful thing. Sometimes it's important, other times it is crucial to understanding. Context can turn villains into heroes.

For fifteen years, I saw death at the doorstep of thousands of people. I waved hello, giving a nod to death as I would with any other work colleague. Death lost its drama—its pizzazz. We became tired foes, having much more in common than we ever realized.

What I'm trying to get at is that there are reasons for what I did. And it's because of context. I want to frame to you what it is an anesthesiologist does so you may begin to understand why I did what I did. After you've read my story I want your conscience to scream to you:

Would I have done the same thing as Jude Rosen?

I THINK it all started with Farrah.

She seemed to be the linchpin in the whole thing.

I usually visited her after work, strangling strangers with my eyes as I chugged along the I-5 North rush-hour slog. Farrah had bunkered down in a cabin on the shores of Whidbey Island. The long drive gave me the unfortunate opportunity to think—to dwell.

I knew Farrah Abdi since undergrad—mean and sarcastic like a beautiful hurricane—exactly why every man in class chased her. I never actually met her until I saw her at a party on campus, told her I noticed her from class. Evidently she'd noticed me, too, as we ended up spending a few moments in a library corner that night. After refusing to recognize my existence in class, we finally got coffee and proceeded to spend the next two years as inseparable idiots. Most weekends were spent blackout drunk with a hangover brunch. We became that reclusive couple that only emerges from our solitary cocoon once every winter solstice. It is still shocking to me that we not only graduated college but with the drunken audacity to get accepted to the same medical school.

Needless to say my parents hated her Iranian guts.

The whole thing ended in a nuclear blowout, of course. Yet I don't think it ever came as a surprise to either one of us. There was unspoken prophecy between us: *This will end poorly. You bring out the drunk in me. I bring out the vilest asshole-of-a-person in you.*

In the fallout of our break-up, a friendship budded like some unkillable cockroach. In medical school, I taught her anatomy while she coached me on mitochondrial diseases, all without sharing another toxic night together. Turned out that by removing the punch-drunk romance, we thrived together and graduated. And like best friends, we did everything else together, including training to become anesthesiologists and working at the same trauma hospital in Seattle. I never would've become a physician without that woman.

Farrah was the love of my life—

One of them.

I STRODE up the muddy path wreathed by brilliant green moss, house keys in hand. She'd had the cabin built on the island a year back, her condo in downtown Seattle now occupied by a new complement of tech bros. I found a sack of unopened groceries on the counter, the stench of dog piss in the air. Her dog Millie found me as I put the groceries away. The dog's leash was lost in the oblivion of the cabin mess so I picked her up and took her to the shore. She took a full minute to empty her bladder.

Farrah's voice issued from the upstairs loft. "Can't keep you away."

"When's the last time you took Millie out?"

"When's the last time you took *Zella* out?" I couldn't see her, but I knew the little shit grin painted on her face.

"You know I house trained Zella years ago."

"True, but accidents can happen to even the best trained wife. I wouldn't judge."

I found her in bed. There was no shit-eating grin. Her face

was skeletal. Thin cords of tendons tented her parchment skin as she groped at the bed covers.

I told her she didn't need to get up.

She cocked an eye at me. "You think I was getting up *for you?* I need to take a shit. Get out!"

I rejoined Millie downstairs and gave her a few pets under the interrupted silence of a diarrheal orchestra.

"I'm ready for you to come wipe my ass now," Farrah beckoned.

"Been waiting my whole life for the honor." She lay in bed once more, her frailness exaggerated by the enormous bed frame. I never knew how so much cynical wrath could be contained in such a tiny body.

She asked me why I had come.

"To torture you further."

"Did your spidey-sense tell you that this was it? That the end was coming?"

"Where has the nurse been? Place looks like shit and I had to throw out the milk that was never put away."

"I fired him."

"You better be joking."

"I'm so *hot*," she said, sitting forward. She lifted her arms like a petulant child and said, "Off."

I helped her off with the shirt, exposing twin scars that swept from her sternum to her armpits. Jagged suture lines cinched the skin like a purse string. Her breasts were rotting away in a pathology lab somewhere.

"That one," she instructed, pointing at a silk robe.

I threw the robe at her face. "Why did you fire the nurse?"

"He was way too attractive."

"Millie hasn't been out in days and the place smells like a pet store. Why would you get rid of the nurse?"

"As if the hospice would actually let me just be here alone. I'm sure another of their stooges will be along any day."

"You can't just…"

"What?"

"You can't just...be here."

"To die alone?"

An ugly silence sat there a moment until she broke it. "I'm serious. He was too young—too damn hot. It was killing me. Making me feel sorry for myself." She sat back in bed and winced.

"How's the pain?" I fiddled through the bevy of prescription bottles on the nightstand.

Methadone. Oxycontin. Oxycodone.

"Bad. It's in my hips and back."

"Are they giving you enough? These are almost empty."

She glared at me a moment as my fingers ran over the prescription bottles. "No. It's not enough. Like taking a sugar pill."

"How are you having so much diarrhea if you're taking this many opiates? You should be backed up as hell."

She only sighed, a film of sweat appearing on her upper lip.

"You must've sweet talked the oncologist pretty good to even get all this prescribed. How could you still be in so much pain? Do you have anything else? Tell me what he's writing for."

She opened her eyes and fixed them on my hands. "Jude."

"What?"

"Put the pills down."

I obeyed, accidentally slamming the bottles on the nightstand, sending pills into the air.

I GOT her down the loft steps and cleared the living room of cardboard boxes and dog food while she called out a neverending list of tasks. Despite the pain, I detected pure joy as her slight frame leaned on a cane, finger pointing at the next chore in the cabin. After vacuuming, I swept the kitchen and washed the dishes which took a good hour since every single plate or utensil was caked with old food. I watered the plants, dusted the blinds and, as the sunlight darkened, cleaned the windows. After she missed the single step from the kitchen and fell, I put her on the couch despite her reassurance that she was fine and to shut the fuck up.

As night fell, we watched Mystery Science Theater 3000 and talked about Spanish pastries and Pearl Jam. She laughed and coughed and then laughed more. We reminisced about eating shawarmas on the corner from our medical school.

It felt good.

It felt young.

It felt like college. Except we skipped the beers.

I hadn't had one in fifteen years.

CHAPTER TWO

Opiates are a beautifully awful thing.

The human body has natural opiates, enkephalins they're called, that release when the body is stressed or in pain. They stimulate pain receptors, modulating the pain response to get the brain to downplay the experience of pain. Because, whether you have a hangnail or a severed arm, pain is all about perception. I've seen a grown man cry like a baby from a needle stick and a little girl get a spinal tap without a peep. Perception is everything. But sometimes, it doesn't matter how tough you are, having a traumatic leg amputation from a motorcycle accident is going to hurt at least a little. And, in that case, natural enkephalins suck at controlling pain.

So without anyone asking, we went ahead and made some improvements.

Most movies show people getting a leg shot full of morphine as they bleed out from an injury. But let's get something clear: morphine is child's play. If you want to continue to writhe in pain *and* itch like hell, then take morphine. If you want to get serious about your painful dismemberment consider dilaudid, oxycodone, hydrocodone, meperidine. When you need something for instant pain relief: fentanyl. Long term chronic cancer pain? Methadone, oxycontin, MS Contin. Anesthesiologists use opiates that other doctors haven't even heard of: remifentanil and sufentanil—drugs that are magnitudes more potent than morphine. And if you're still in pain, I'm happy to give you a dash of ketamine to clean up after the opiates. Anesthesiologists carry the most powerful narcotics known to humankind in the front pocket of our scrubs. Sometimes when I bend over to tie my shoe, they fall on the floor—thousands of street dollars just looking up at me.

Hello, they say. Hello.

Opiates are beautiful because they work. They're also awful...because they work. When used briefly and appropriately, opiates are mana. When used longer than a few days, they send you walking through the valley of death. Yes, you'll get pain relief after your car accident but you might leave the hospital with an addiction. Back in the 90s and early 2000s, pain doctors dished out opiates to their patients with chronic pain, turning up millions of dollars. Turns out, however, when your brain wants to stop taking them, your body tells you *nope*. The age of synthetic opiates created droves of new addicts—Americans that would've never even heard the word 'fentanyl' in their entire white-bread lives. And now, in the age of the opiate crisis, we tell those same patients that we're sorry, but we can't be your drug dealer anymore. So then they go find Shane or Scud or Scar or Zach at the gas station to score them a dime bag.

You're welcome, America.

I KEEP them in a metal lock box that I secure to my anesthesia cart with a lock and key. It's a cornucopia of narcotics: fentanyl, dilaudid and midazolam—five vials each. I use this box throughout my day at work, keeping them close and on demand to administer to patients while they're on the operating table. When you're about to faint from nerves as I bring you to the OR—midazolam. It'll make you feel about three beers deep. When your heart rate spikes as the surgeon drives a scalpel through the abdomen—fentanyl. Your reflexes will chill out. When you wake up in agony after a neurosurgeon fixed your spine with twelve screws—dilaudid. You'll forget where you are. And if you still have problems, hell I'll stick a bag of the stuff to your IV and you can press a button any time you want a hit.

For those that have never taken an opiate in their lives, pain control is a piece of cake. A dash of fentanyl and a bolus of dilaudid will take care of you. The challenge is with those whose veins are already saturated with the stuff—the addicts and the chronic pain people. Their bodies develop this funny little thing called tolerance.

Tolerance.

In most cases, a good thing, but not when it comes to opiates. When your body tolerates opiates it means all those cute little receptors start downregulating because they know there is plenty of the drug in the bloodstream, so they try to decrease the degree of stimulation. This makes the next dose less effective...and the next dose less effective...and the next dose less effective. And for those addicts out there, it makes the next high less effective...and the next high less effective...and the next high less effective—

You need more.

More. And more and more.

And after you have more, you need a dump truck brimming with vicodin, percocet and oxycontin to dump the payload directly into your mouth. That will tide you over for about an hour until your next fix. And the absolute hilarious thing about tolerance is that it makes you tolerant to all of opiate effects *except the ones that will actually kill you.* Meaning, as your body gets less of a high every time you increase the dose, your brain will still tell your lungs to stop breathing as you escalate the dose.

This is how people die.

You inject more and more, trying to find that original high yet it gets less and less gratifying. But all along, the respiratory depression increases by the same degree until you give yourself that one...

Final.

Dose.

So, I keep them in a metal box, locked to the top of my anesthesia cart. A grab bag of the world's most powerful narcotics at my fingertips. I draw them up in a syringe and keep them handy in my pocket like a neat little line of pens.

Would they have handed me the keys to this box had they known about me? Would they have admitted me to anesthesia residency knowing all the binge drinking weekdays with Farrah in college? Would they have admitted us *both?*

I was a walking redflag.

But me and Farrah were smart, could pass some tests—a lot of tests—without being too brainy and on-the-spectrum during job interviews. Medical schools want well rounded people—not a savant who doesn't know how to carry a conversation. At any rate, I'd made it as a physician with the sneaking suspicion that I was a fraud. I was able to check all the academic boxes and meet whatever clandestine criteria admission committees kept, whether that was throwing a dart at a board or something with more metrics, I never knew.

But, how can they really know who they've accepted into the profession? How do you know if you're recruiting the Craigslist Killer or Doctor Death? How do you know that you can trust someone with stockpiles of the world's most potent narcotics?

Most of the time, the system of creating doctors works. Chances are, if you have the tenacity to actually make it through all that education, you're likely going to be an upstanding citizen who can be trusted. 99.9% of the time, you can trust your anesthesiologist to monitor your sedated and paralyzed body. But there's always that 0.1%. That one vulnerable window where your anesthesiologist just isn't having his or her best day.

And maybe, that's the one day you need an operation.

"CODE BLUE" was announced overhead as my pager blared the same message. I was groggy from my late drive back from Farrah's—my five year old, Kris, crying about robbers in her room also didn't help.

I stopped running to Codes Blues, long ago.

I realized the one minute of time that I saved by sprinting to a Code in the hospital had to be made up with another minute of catching my breath. I also learned the sometimes total and complete futility of all our medical efforts when someone is dying. That can decentivize you. So I walked, drugs in my front pocket, airway bag in hand. There was no hurry to watch someone die.

In the emergency department, I elbowed my way through the crowd of med students and nurses and got to the head of the bed where a woman groaned, her face white as a sheet of paper. EMS was spouting history: she was found down, half a liter blood loss, bullet wound in her neck—

Bullet wound in the neck. That got my interest.

She groaned—usually a sign of life. I found the wound just in from the carotid and jugular. Miraculously the bullet missed the major vessels otherwise she'd have bled out already. As I wondered if her trachea had been punctured, she answered a resounding *yes* as she coughed up a spoonful of blood. With her pulse oximeter in the mid-eighties, I knew she had at least one lungful of blood. She needed a secure airway, fast.

I drew up medications:

Rocuronium to reversibly paralyze the body: can't have a person choking and flailing while I'm shoving a breathing tube down their throat. Fentanyl to blunt the fight-or-flight reflexes: can't have their heart rate and blood pressure sky high as I rake on the vocal cords. Propofol for sedation: can't have you suing me for awareness while you are fully paralyzed with instrumentation in your mouth. It's not an experience you want to remember. Fortunately her blood pressure was still normal as I slammed in the meds. Her body turned off in 9.8 seconds so I hinged her forehead back, scissored open the mouth and inserted the anesthesiologist's best friend:

The laryngoscope.

Fancy name for handle with a dull, metal blade.

Usually when you advance the blade past the teeth, past the tongue and into the recesses of the throat—if you're doing things right—you see the beautiful vocal cords staring back at you, begging for you to place a breathing tube.

I saw nothing but blood.

Pools of blood, sheets of blood. Geysers of blood coming from within the trachea.

"Suction!" I yelled.

Double suction was placed in the mouth, and for a moment, I thought things would improve. But once the blood cleared, all I saw was swollen tissue completely crowding the airway and I immediately knew what had happened. The bullet had caused a hematoma—a collection of blood—within the facial tissues, completely distorting the airway. I could hear the pulse ox without looking, the tone dropping low as if accompanying the symphony of my struggle. There was no way I was going to get a clear view of the vocal cords with my laryngoscope.

"Fiberoptic!" I yelled.

A moment later, someone placed a fiberoptic camera in my fingers—an oblong handle equipped with knobs and levers, a thin tail attached to the end like a whip—a small camera mounted with a light, projecting the image on a screen to my left. I threaded the camera through her mouth and plunged it into the pool of blood, broadcasting nothing but darkness on the screen. I pushed gingerly, blindly navigating the swollen tissue until I felt a release. The screen showed scattered light through a fleshy tunnel. My camera was in one of two places: the trachea—good—or the esophagus—bad.

Her pulse ox was low—very low.

Her heart rate was low—very low.

I heard the ER doc yell, "Secure the airway!"

Not sure what she thought I was currently doing.

As I swiveled the fiberoptic camera, I thought I saw rings

of tracheal cartilage so I railroaded a breathing tube over the fiberoptic, pulled out the camera and hooked a ventilator up to the tube—

I was in the trachea—

Maybe.

As I squeezed the ventilator, I saw her chest rise as oxygen filled her lungs. The pulse ox chirped with a high tone and her heart rate started to pick up. I looked over at the surgeon who had been watching. "Hope you like digging for lead." I pushed the bed toward the operating rooms.

"HOW DID THAT CASE GO?" Someone called behind me.

But it wasn't just someone. It was Lazlo. Not for lack of a better word, he was my boss—chief of anesthesia staff. There were many other words I would prefer to describe him, but boss was the kindest. He always furrowed his eyebrows at me as if concerned out of pity—something he'd done since day one of my residency. He shed the condescension for residents when they were hired on as staff anesthesiologists—except for me. Fifteen years I'd been dealing with the man. Don't people retire? Or die off?

I told him the case went fine and turned to leave.

"Jude, have you checked your narc lock box?"

"No, why?"

"It's still in your OR. Wide open."

Shit. I'd forgotten to lock my narcotic lock box after the case. Something about suctioning blood from the woman's lungs while the surgeons dug around in her neck for four hours had me distracted. I told him I'd take care of it but he set those furrowed eyebrows on me. "It's an easy way to lose opiates," he told me, "you don't want to lose track of those, do you?"

He was right, of course. Tedious and careful record keeping must be kept by every anesthesiologist of their narcotic use throughout the day. The narc lock boxes are stocked every morning by pharmacists and placed in a locked, automatic dispensary. My fingerprint gained access and tracked the exact narc box that was taken. Throughout the day, as I gave the narcotics to patients in the OR, I charted the administration in the medical health record. At the end of the day, I noted what was used and left the surplus back in the narc box to be locked up again. This way, any pharmacist could come along and audit my narcotic use to check for discrepancy. One discrepancy once in a year could be explained by an anesthesiologist being forgetful of charting. Pharmacy watched you like a hawk. Multiple discrepancies and you had a urine drug test coming your way and maybe even a visit from the DEA. I know because it happened to me during residency. The urine drug screening anyways, didn't quite have to get the DEA involved.

"I said I'll take care of it," I told Lazlo and turned to leave again.

He then asked, "How is she?"

I set my jaw. "Alive."

I found my narc box back in the OR, the box wide open. The vials looked up at me, nothing disturbed.

Hello, they said. Hello.

A FEW DAYS LATER, I visited Farrah again, told her that Lazlo was concerned enough to ask about her.

"Always the saint," she said, a grimace on her face. She lay in bed, sweat coating her forehead, breathing fast. She was in pain. More than usual. "Does he think you're diverting?"

Diverting.

It was a nice word for an anesthesiologist who was stealing narcs, either for personal use or for street sale. When I started residency, they taught us the signs: wearing long sleeves in the OR to cover track marks, chaotic personal life, wanting more time alone in the OR to divert. It was rare but more common than you'd think. They said one in one hundred anesthesiology residents was diverting and abusing. "It could happen to anyone. It could happen to you," they said.

I didn't believe it until I saw it.

A Code Blue was called one night during my residency. I ran with the team, my airway bag around my shoulder, eager to put a breathing tube into someone. Instead of running toward the patient wards—where actual patients were—the Code Blue team was led to a dark hallway in the basement.

The physician call rooms.

I remember the confusion: what was a dying patient doing in the doctor call rooms? Of course when we came into the call room, the awful reality of everything crashed over our heads: the Code Blue was for a physician. Doctor Kara, an anesthesiologist, lay stiff and motionless—a needle at her side.

I just stared at her blue lips.

It could happen to anyone. It could happen to you.

I didn't believe it until I saw her there.

I didn't believe it until it happened to me.

"No, he doesn't think I'm diverting. He's just being Lazlo," I told Farrah.

She shot me a sidelong look. "Because you're...*not* diverting?"

I was actually hurt. Which is something only she could do. "You think I wouldn't tell you?"

She slowly nodded. It was annoying. "It's been twelve years. Addictions don't care about time."

I clenched my fists—genuine anger. "I will *never* do it again."

"Is that because you're such a different person now? Everything has changed?" Her eyes were pearly orbs, wet and ominous within the sag of her eyelids.

I knew she was pushing me—testing me—but it still pissed me off. "You want me to say that I could relapse?"

"I want you to respect the addiction. Respect it as the parasite that it is."

I was both mad and grateful. She wouldn't bring it up if she didn't care. "I know."

"It will always be with you. And the moment you think it's gone—bam!" She clapped her hands, genuinely startling me. "It will bite again."

At that moment, I loved her so much. Not the rabid, hurricane relationship we had in college but the patient love that only a true friend can bear. Farrah rescued me. She saved me, back then during residency, she saved me from myself. Soon after I saw Doctor Kara, rigor mortis setting in—I was diverting and injecting myself. I used my feet veins—my shoes covered up the track marks. I was fast tracked to become the next Code Blue.

It was all so stupidly tragic and obvious.

But Farrah knew—she knew me to the core. She took away the fentanyl, took away the needles. She provided me with a fresh cup of her own urine so I could pass the test when Lazlo was on to me. She saved me from the parasite and, along with it, saved my life and career.

"I love you," I told her, taking her emaciated hand in mine.

"If you love me, don't go back. Not ever." She barely spoke as she chased a worried look from her face. Dread crept within her like a shadow. There was a deep worry there. Cancer pain was settling into her bones, burrowing in, making a home.

"Never," I said, "never again."

I wasn't lying.

CHAPTER THREE

I had a wife throughout all this.

Zella.

The other love of my life. And don't worry, this isn't a story about an affair. I *wish* it were a story about an affair.

An affair was better than what really happened.

ZELLA WAS WELL aware of my visits with Farrah and joined me on more than one occasion. Zella, too, had a set of keys to Farrah's cabin and visited her often, cleaning and bringing cookies that she wouldn't eat. As much as Farrah made fun of her, she loved Zella but not because of what she did for her, but for what Zella did for me. She kept me on even keel—she was the ship to which I'd been hitched. Zella was the reason why I didn't lie to Farrah that I would never go back. With her as my wife, I had all the borrowed strength I would need. Farrah did all the dirty work of fixing me and Zella took me the rest of the way from self-destruction. When Zella came into my life, it was a white lightning bolt of such earnest and wholesome intent that I could never get her out of my mind.

There was no one like her.

Before I knew she existed, I was still in residency—weeks after my last diversion and use. It was only recently that Lazlo was onto me—certain that I was using—and Farrah had vouched for me. Farrah, my resident classmate who handed me a cup of clean urine and put me on her own rehab course—The Six Week Recovery for Jude. I slipped past the stooges in pharmacy, past Lazlo, and past expulsion and getting my medical license revoked.

It was on the heels of my secret recovery when I was in the neuro ICU as a resident. There were four kinds of patients there: those who got a small whack on the head—a minor brain bleed who left the ICU in a couple days. There were the ones who had a ticking time bomb of an aneurysm that finally exploded, coating their brain with caustic blood that spasmed their major arteries, causing strokes. A select few had fallen into a fate worse than death: locked in. The patient is conscious, but completely paralyzed. The only way we know someone is still in there is blink once for no, twice for yes. The last group of patients were those who got hit so hard on the head their brains swelled up and herniated through their spinal cords. Brain death. Or in other words—death. Trying to explain to families that their loved one is dead when they still have a pulse is not necessarily straightforward. It was a sad place. It was during a time when I was still naive enough to be saddened by sickness.

The patients were mostly comatose, breathing tube in place, ventilator pumping their lungs. Because of their coma or sedation, the patients were easy to reduce down to physiological components: heart rate high? Give X. Blood pressure low?

Give Y. Septic shock? Shotgun spectrum of antibiotics. One of the necessary skills of being a physician is also an inherent flaw in the profession: separate the humanity from the work—compartmentalize patients into mechanical components. And can you blame us? Can you really expect us to process a dozen human tragedies a day and go home to our families with a smile on our faces? Does anyone really wonder why physician suicide rate is one of the highest of all professions?

I had a patient with spasm of the blood vessels of the brain—a young woman. She had lost the genetic lottery and had an aneurysm at birth which blew out while she was water skiing. For days she lay in bed, breathing on her own—no interaction. She stared and blinked and had bowel movements.

With each passing day I rounded on her, wrote orders, and moved onto the next patient. And every day, she stared and she blinked. She became a mirror—a reflection of futility. Why was she there, in that bed, and I wasn't? Did it even make a difference? Every day I saw her, I thought about diverting narcotics. She lay slumped in bed, more and more, until she became almost amorphous—a vague shape of a human being wrapped in blankets. I knew she'd never wake up again. Oh, she'd live, but she would get shipped off to a nursing home to live out her days with a feeding tube in her gut. But on her tenth day in the hospital, something was radically different about her.

She smiled at me.

She was up, sitting out of bed, while a nurse was shampooing her hair. I watched as the nurse rinsed her long hair into a basin, dried it, gave a brief scalp massage and then proceeded to brush out the tangles. The nurse chatted her up like they were at a hair salon, the patient laughing and talking about her family.

I was totally floored.

Shampooing and brushing a patient's hair is not in a nurse's job description.

The patient recovered, not because of any medicine or therapy I gave her, but because a nurse dignified her as a human being—helping clear the patient's delirium.

Quickly, I found out the nurse's name.

I observed Zella that week—saw how she interacted with patients. Everyone was a friend, every person was a human being, *not* a fleshy bag of organ systems to treat. She chatted with them, ate lunch with them and ushered their families in to visit at any time of day. I realized that she was how a healthcare worker was supposed to behave. I'd probably crossed her path a hundred times but never really noticed her, thinking her too plain. She was the reason that I probably wanted to be in medicine to begin with—to help people.

Novel idea.

AND SHE WAS INCREDIBLE, amazing—all the superlatives I can think of.

The love story for me and Zella is as basic as love stories get. So basic and beautiful that to fully recount it would reduce us down to a cliché. I noticed her, she noticed me and things went from there. All along, I kept a distance, knowing she was someone I shouldn't be with—couldn't be with. Yet that drew her in. I was guarded for months until she dragged it out of me—my problems with alcohol, problems with diverting narcotics. I thought for sure she'd be done with me—that it would be the end of the story.

But she was the beginning of a new story.

Farrah brought me up from the quicksand, but Zella—she

kept me from falling back. She kept me afloat with a loyalty and dedication that dumbfounded me then and forever. Zella was a foundry of compassion, the most of which she inexplicably reserved for me. I felt bad at the time—thought I knew why she wanted to be with me. That I was the project, the guy that she could finally make better. All of that was true, of course, but she was right—she could fix me, make me better. And I was better. Never once while being with Zella did I think about putting another toxic substance into my body.

But maybe a person is only good because of the people that surround them. You take them away, and what do you have? I'd thought for the past fifteen years that I *was* different, that my family *had* changed me. But maybe people are no more complex than lab rats—they behave according to the stimulus of their environment. Give a food pellet and all is well. Give a shock and—

They revert to more primal instincts.

WE LIVED a little outside the city, bordering rural. It was a pain to commute to the hospital across Lake Washington everyday, but we liked the space. Our neighbors were exactly how you like them: dull and quiet. Even our next door neighbor, some young guy with the inexplicably enormous home, barely made a noise except for the occasional party.

Zella always wanted a greenhouse, so we built a greenhouse. She wanted fresh parsley and cucumbers, so we grew them. She wanted two children, so we had them.

"But why though, Dad, why?" Regina asked.

My daughter was nine. Smart and everything annoying that comes with being precocious. "I don't know. I don't know why spiders have book lungs. I don't even know what book lungs are." I couldn't answer half the questions she threw at me.

"Mites don't have them. Even though they're arachnids."

I nodded, eating, shaking off the day.

"How is she?" Zella asked from across the table, bouncing our five-year-old, Kris, on her lap. The girl had proceeded to chew and regurgitate broccoli into her palm.

I said, "Couldn't get her out of bed."

Regina leaned in her chair. "Are you talking about Aunt Farrah?"

"Yes."

"Why not?" Zella asked.

"The pain is everywhere."

"Doesn't she have meds?"

"Yes. Boat loads. And I watch her take them."

Zella sighed, wiping Kris' mouth. "I'll go see her tomorrow."

"You don't need to. She got a new nurse. Finally."

"Can we have her down here this weekend? Dinner?"

I imagined trying to get Farrah's tiny body out of that cabin and into a car. "I doubt it."

"Does she have any upcoming appointments at the hospital?"

I lifted my face from dinner. "There's nothing else for her to do there."

"Are you being a doomy gloomy daddy?" Regina asked.

I shrugged.

"Mom, can we fix doomy gloomy daddy?" she asked Zella.

Zella smiled. "Tomorrow, we'll go."

WE WENT TO THE PARK.

Watching Regina help little Kris up a plastic slide was a balm to my doomy gloomy soul. I collected the gloom, like a dark sponge from work and needed a periodic wringing. All the motor vehicle traumas, drug addicts with flesh-eating bacterial infections, the execution-style gang shootings and the young people with noose markings around their necks—it was some sort of macabre merry-go-round for me. I always told myself I was desensitized—that it didn't affect me. But seeing my own little girls playing, skipping, jumping—there was a release of the doomy gloomy. I unwittingly bottled it up through the week and they helped me get it out—to process the mass human tragedy.

The innocence of the children was bright to me. It filled me with something more than the deep rooted fatalism that almost had a stranglehold on me during the week. It was the same feeling when I saw Zella the first time, brushing that woman's hair. They—my girls—were why I didn't slip back, why I didn't relapse into who I was.

Yet on that Saturday, the darkness wouldn't leave me.

"It's Farrah," Zella said, taking her hand in mine.

I nodded. She always knew.

"What can we do for her?"

"There's nothing."

She gripped my hand. "There's always something. What can we *do* for her?"

I let go of her hand and thought on that a long while.

WE WENT to a Salvation Army and riffled through the board games. Miraculously I found an old video-cassette based game, Atmosfear, where a demon on tape would guide players through the horrors of a board game. Farrah and I played it with friends in college. I knew it was hard for Zella, watching my face light up as I reminisced about an old girlfriend. But she cared about me and she loved Farrah which absolved her of the petty emotions of which most people suffer. We bought snacks, packed a kayak on the car and headed for Whidbey Island.

After suffering the I-5 slog, we arrived at Farrah's cabin. I put my key in the lock, the door opened inward to the frown of a stranger.

"Can I help you?" the woman said, the frown lines never disappearing from her mouth.

I resisted the urge to laugh at the woman and move her aside but said, "We're here to visit Farrah."

"She does not want visitors."

"And you are?"

She folded burly arms over her chest. "Her new hospice nurse. She just told me now. No visitors."

"I'm not a visitor. Tell her Jude and Zella are here."

"She knows you're here. She still says no." The nurse moved to close the door.

"But—"

"She's very ill. Does not want visitors."

"And she knows it's us? With the kids?"

She nodded. "Please. Leave."

The door closed.

MUCH LATER THAT night after the disquiet and confusion from Farrah's new nurse, I heard Zella whisper something to me. Beneath the covers of our bed, I couldn't hear.

"What?" I asked her, moving toward her side of the bed.

She didn't turn, didn't open her eyes. She repeated, "It's okay you still love her."

"It's not like that."

"Are you sure?"

"I love her but...not like that anymore. Not for a long time."

"You'd tell me?"

"I would tell you anything."

"You promise?"

"Yes."

CHAPTER FOUR

Days later, at work, it felt like the weekend didn't happen. The therapy from my kids at the park, Zella—evaporated. I was the angry troll at work: short with medical students who didn't shut up and impatient with residents who took a million years to do anything. I must've appeared a tremendous asshole. And I was one, too. It wasn't even a busy day. I wasn't on trauma duty. I was doing something much worse:

Colonoscopies.

I've painted anesthesiology as a neck-breaking thrill ride, but it isn't like that everyday. Anesthesiologists are also the doctors of comfort. When a person might feel one modicum of discomfort during any procedure whatsoever, an anesthesiologist is consulted. There are thousands of procedures done in a hospital. Some entail digging a bullet out of a trachea, others involve putting a camera up someone's butt. We run the whole gambit of stabilizing patients and sometimes it's the difference between life and death and other times it's the difference between life and—

Paint drying.

At times we're just a seismograph: a boring box with a tiny needle calibrated by some arcane academic and placed in the corner of a basement of a faceless government building. We sit, we wait, we watch and we monitor. No one really notices the seismograph—you don't even think about it. A little fentanyl or midazolam, dash of propofol, and you're going to be comfortable while a gastroenterologist puts anything in your body, below or above. Yet, even in that anesthetic, there is an inherent danger. In the world of anesthesiology, boredom is lethal.

Having vigilance of danger in the face of boredom is one of the hardest things about the job. Most of the time, boredom is a good thing for patients. When your anesthesiologist is bored, it means everything is going fine—that there is nothing exciting enough to occupy our attention. But when that boredom starts lending to inattention, that's when the anesthesiologist doesn't notice that you've become so oversedated that you're no longer protecting your airway. That's when you vomit and aspirate half a liter into your lungs. Many Code Blues started with just a simple sedation—a little procedure—that turned into chest compressions.

So, doing an entire day full of colonoscopies is not my favorite. It's high turnover, meaning I'm doing eight to ten cases in a row, moving and pushing drugs all day while intermittently watching a camera screen broadcasting someone's rectum to the room. It's both busy and dull.

After a day of colonoscopies, I was doing eyeballs. Cataract babysitting or retinal reattachment—only slightly less exciting than doing colonoscopies. The next day I was assigned to the hand room—blocking the nerves to a patient's hand enough so they can't feel cuts or pin placements. They get just enough propofol to keep them lightly sedated. A monkey could do the anesthetic. The next day I was in breast flap reconstruction surgery—basically watching a plastic surgeon make microscopic blood vessel repairs for about ten hours while I sit on a stool and monitor vitals. The boredom was killing me and I was itching to be back in the trauma bay. That evening I looked at my assignment posted for the next day—colonoscopies.

Again.

I called after him down the hallway. “Lazlo.” He looked at me with those expectant, baleful eyes. Always full of pity or something—a reproachful distrust. Something I could never put my finger on but loathed nonetheless. “What’s up with the rooms you’re putting me in?”

He gazed at me, maintaining an innocent musing. “What do you mean?”

“Been bored out of my mind all week. You usually split up the stool-sitting cases amongst everyone—spreading the joy. Put me back on trauma.”

He cleared his throat. A bad sign. “There have been complaints.”

“Okay...Put me back on trauma.”

“That bloody airway you did last week. The surgeons and ER staff didn’t like your behavior—didn’t like how you barked out orders and then took the patient to the operating room without the surgeons input first.”

“Uh huh. And how’s the patient doing?”

“Fine.”

“Not just fine. She’s home. She left the hospital completely healthy today. Do you think she would be alive if she continued to bleed into her airway? Do you think anyone had any idea what was going on until I showed up?”

"There are protocols to follow."

"Do you think that patient gave a shit about your protocols?"

A painfully awkward pause cropped up.

Good. I wanted it there.

He put his hand on my shoulder. "I think you need to cool off for a few days in some easy rooms."

I backed up, his hand flapping away. "I've done enough rectal punishment for not playing nice. Just put me on trauma tomorrow."

THE NEXT DAY I looked at the OR board and there I was, scheduled for colonoscopies. I suppressed the anger and unlocked my narc box from the pharmacy locker. As the colonoscopies slogged by that morning, I flinched with every trauma code that was called overhead. I knew the anesthesiologist on trauma duty that day, Dr. Cappe. He was a decent chap but could barely figure out where to stick a breathing tube. Who the hell knew what kind of ass-backward things were going on in the ER?

As I wheeled out my fourth colonoscopy patient to the recovery room, yet another trauma code blared from the overhead speaker. I blurted out the colonoscopy case details to the recovery nurse: patient had a little midazolam, a little propofol, still sleepy but will likely wake up soon—

I was interrupted by the overhead operator uttering the most beautiful words to an anesthesiologist: "Surgical airway, stat, to the Emergency Department."

Surgical. Airway.

There's a lot of information loaded into those two words. It means someone has tried to put a breathing tube into a patient but has either failed so badly that they've swelled the airway beyond recognition or that the patient's airway is so messed up to begin with that you don't even know where to put the tube.

Without another word, I left the nurse there with my patient, twirling around a gurney moving at me. The nurse yelled something about having to start the next case. Not only did I not care about starting the next colonoscopy on time, I knew Dr. Cappe wouldn't have the first clue about doing a surgical airway down in the ER.

The ER was a riot of bustling nurses and paramedics. I clamored to the main resuscitation bay and saw a dogpile of healthcare workers floundering over a massive patient, limbs and head sprawled over the gurney. Everyone was doing something but none of it seemed to be helping the acutely blue patient dying in front of them. The pulse ox was in the fifties and the heart rate was...there—but not for long. I saw Cappe at the head of the bed, face frozen in a grimace of nothing but white, sweaty fear. His arms flailed with a laryngoscope in one hand and a fiberoptic camera in another—he was trying everything under the sun to secure the airway. I put my hands on the patient's thigh. He was warm—way too warm. I then realized everything about the patient was exaggerated, facial features bloated, hands blown up like balloons—

Anaphylaxis.

Whatever it was that had made the man swell up, the same thing was happening in the airway. There was no way Cappe was going to get a breathing tube from above.

"Surgical airway tray!" I yelled while elbowing my way to the head of the bed.

Relief flashed across Cappe's face when he saw me. He put down his instruments in frustration while the pulse ox beeped lower and lower, down into dead man's territory. "It's impossible," he declared.

I didn't say anything as I splashed iodine on the patient's neck, the maroon liquid flying over everyone. The pager at my waist beeped and vibrated for my attention, something of which I had little at the moment. So I ripped open the surgical tray kit and immediately found what I was looking for: a single needle and syringe. With needle in right hand, I palpated the patient's neck, feeling for the trachea. Amongst the boggy flesh, it may as well have been a thousand miles deep. I dug deeper with my fingertips, feeling for some anatomical landmark but there was nothing. I ignored the patient's blue lips, his glassy eyes glued on the ceiling—oblivious now to the surrounding struggle. The heart rate was beeping way too low—that was it, cardiac arrest was coming any second. I could finally feel the trachea, but didn't know where I was along its length. If I put the needle in too low I could collapse a lung—too much to the left or right and I'd puncture the thyroid or carotids, potentially causing massive bleeding.

He was dead, anyway.

So I dug the needle into his neck, pulling back on the syringe as I advanced. Nothing...nothing...nothing—and then I felt a release of air into the syringe. It meant my needle had made its way into the trachea—probably. I removed the syringe, leaving the needle in place, and then grabbed a wire, feeding one end in. The wire threaded smoothly and the patient bucked as it went down into his lungs—that was good. It meant his brain reflexes were still intact.

With wire in place, I took out the needle, shoved a skin dilator around the wire and then threaded a tracheostomy tube over the wire. With the trach in place, I whipped out the wire and hooked up a ventilator bag and started pumping air. While holding my breath I waited for that one sweet vital sign to pop up on the monitor:

Carbon dioxide.

It's the gold standard to know if you have successfully placed a breathing tube in the right place. And there they were —those beautiful waveform tracings of carbon dioxide, rising and falling with each breath. The patient's pulse ox chirped up along with the heart rate.

Cappe looked at me with a dumbass smile and the entire room exhaled a collective sigh of relief. I turned and saw the ENT surgeons standing there, looking at me.

I told them, "Little too late, boys and girls," and slapped one of them on the back. It was an asshole move that I may have relished just a little bit.

They weren't happy.

FEELING ENTIRELY SATISFIED WITH MYSELF, I mosied back upstairs to colonoscopy detention. I discovered my previous patient, the one I'd left with the recovery nurse, had somehow gotten a breathing tube.

I looked at the nurse, mouth ajar in disbelief. "What happened?"

"We were paging you," she said, an edge in her voice.

"Why? What was wrong?"

She went on to explain that the patient's airway was obstructing, that they couldn't wake her up, that her pulse ox was in the 80s.

"So?" I told her, "you give a little jaw thrust, open up the airway or you put in an oral airway until she perks up. Who put that tube in?"

"I did," someone said behind me. But I already knew it was Lazlo.

"*Why?*"

"Where were you?" he asked.

"Downstairs, helping with the surgical airway. Why does this patient have a breathing tube?"

"You were supposed to be supervising the recovery unit. Why did you leave?"

"I already told you, to help with the surgical airway. It was a total shit show down there." My voice was rising, something I was usually good at keeping cool.

"Dr. Cappe was on trauma duty, not you."

"Dr. Cappe was standing over a blue, dying patient before I showed up down there."

"That doesn't matter. Because you left, you weren't here to supervise the recovery room and the nursing staff had to call me in to intubate this patient."

I'm not easily dumbfounded, but the guy had me. "You didn't need to put a tube in, she just needed more time to wake up. Now thanks to you, she's going to spend a night in the intensive care unit."

"Not because of me—because of you, not doing the job you were assigned to do."

"But you could've just given her a jaw thrust, *not* put in a tube."

"No, *you* could've done that. Not me." He turned, done with me.

I watched him walk away, there was a hint of swagger in his walk.

I GOT HOME THAT NIGHT, grateful it was a Friday and that I

wasn't working the weekend. Zella had left earlier with the kids for pizza. Farrah was on my mind. I wondered what she was doing—wondered if she was even alive. Maybe she had died that day, while I was cutting into someone's airway and bringing them back from the brink. Farrah could've been traded out. She was so frail at that point, that her death would've been just a little wink—a small light turning off. She wasn't close to her family, most of whom were still in Iran. No one would notice or be with her as she shuffled off.

Why did she send me away?

Zella discovered me on the couch, sitting there in a dark room, brooding about Farrah and festering over Lazlo.

"Should we garden tomorrow?" she asked, her hand sliding down my back. I knew it was supposed to be comforting. I didn't want to be comforted.

"Sure."

"Sure means no."

I said nothing.

Regina looked at me, mouth puckered. "Dad's not going to hang out tonight, is he?"

How could I tell her? How could I explain to my little girl what my day had been like? She could never know. "Not tonight," I told her. I wasn't strong enough to bring her into my lap, play games or turn on a movie. None of that was going to happen tonight. It would've been a time like that where I'd want a beer, or I would've diverted something from work—but those demons had fled long ago.

At least I thought they had.

Respect the addiction. Respect it as the cunning parasite that it is.

Farrah's eyes—her voice, reminding me of everything that I'd overcome.

"I'm sorry," I finally said to my girls. I always wished I could've been better for them. I'd never felt like a real husband or a real father. There was someone in my mind pointing a finger down at me: *you're no doctor, you're no husband, you're no father.*

You are a fraud.

And that was the real demon. Not the booze or the opiates —it was the self-doubt, the certainty that I didn't belong where I was. But wait—I'd saved a man that day, hadn't I? He would've died without me? And wait—I have a wife, she wouldn't love me if I didn't have something redeeming about me, right? And thus marched on the brain of Jude Rosen. This was my cycle, over and over—self-doubt, surrender, toxic habit, someone pulls me up, I turn into an arrogant asshole. It used to be Farrah who got me out of the cycle.

But now it was Zella.

She could see the gears of my human condition churning in my dumb brain. And she waited. And she waited. She swept a tear from my eye and said, "Where is Kojak?"

Our black lab. "I thought he was with you," I said.

Regina shook her head. "Did you lose Kojak, dad?" Even my daughter talked to me like I was a total screw up.

"Hey." Zella shook her head at Regina. "Sometimes he just gets out of the yard."

I went to the door, shoving my feet into running shoes and shrugging on a jacket. "I'll go find him."

I yelled the dog's name down the street but with no moon and crickets blaring, I couldn't see or hear a thing. I went across the street, knocked on the neighbor's door but no one answered. I looked back at our house and then to our next door neighbor—the enormous mansion owned by some young guy with a face and a name that I couldn't pick out of a lineup of one. I'd never actually met the guy who rarely seemed to be home but I thought I'd give him a try.

YOU SOMETIMES HEAR stories or movies about one event—one train missed or one airplane that arrived late—and it completely changed someone's life. We think these stories are nonsense, that you are who you are and no mundane event is going to be life altering. I never gave such mysticism a thought but I never would've supposed that losing a dog would be a major, earth-shattering branching point in my life, either. What would've happened if Kojak hadn't gotten out that night?

I don't ask these questions anymore.

Not only because they're stupid questions but mostly because they don't matter.

CHAPTER FIVE

So I walked up the steps to our next door neighbor's home and knocked. The guy opened. Skinny, white, late 20s with a terrible goatee. He was shirtless with a beaded necklace around his neck—empty eyes as if looking at the horizon. Before I could open my mouth, he reached out two fingers and touched my lips as if to silence me. "Pppfft!" I backed up, wiping my lips with the back of my hand. "What're you *doing*?"

He lowered his dirty fingers and then gave a deep bow. "Enter." He twirled with a flourish of his arms and disappeared inside his home.

"I'm just looking for my dog," I yelled from the porch, "black lab. Have you seen him?"

My only answer was the stench of weed, wafting from within.

His voice finally bounced around the foyer. "I haven't seen your dog, Doctor Rosen."

"We've met?" We probably had and I just didn't remember. Happened to me all the time with people.

"No. Why don't you come in. It's your lucky day, I have blueberries and coconut water. They'll help you."

I don't know why I walked into the guy's house. I normally don't socialize, especially with people I don't know—it's just exhausting as hell. But there was something about the guy's informality—a familiarity that put me at ease.

His house was a palace. Full of multi-storied platforms showcasing crystal animal statues—some in sex poses—stringed instruments crafted in countries I couldn't pronounce and colorful tribal masks. He must've bought some stoner, shaman starter package on eBay. It was all very worthy of a good eye roll and an excuse to go home. But when I saw him standing in the kitchen, a massive bowl of blueberries in hand, I pulled up a stool. I had him pegged. He was the type that loved to outrage and was only intrigued when someone was totally unphased. I was game.

"I felt it right when I opened the door," he explained. "Your throat chakra is tight as a wind-up toy. You can't get anything out." He looked down at me over his wire glasses.

"Been meaning to get that looked at."

He craned his neck back, a succinct laugh erupted from his throat. "You've come to the right place. Eat."

I ate the blueberries with the guy. We munched in silence. It was weird.

I explained more about the dog, shared the acceptable pleasantries of social etiquette (where you from originally, we'll have you over for dinner sometime and so forth) and got up to leave, not entirely sorry that I met the guy.

"Come here," he said, ignoring the social cues of someone trying to get the hell out of there. He lifted his hands toward my face. "I can help you. Let me be a good neighbor."

"Help with what?" He looked at me all cock-eyed and

sassy. I wasn't sure of his sexual orientation but based on the decor, he could've been into anything. I certainly did not want to give him the wrong idea. I told him I needed to find the dog but he came right up to me, holding his hands close to my throat.

"Close your eyes."

Intrigued by the novelty of this new person in my life, I did as told.

"Now," he said in the tone of a yoga instructor, "imagine there is a spool of thread at your throat. The thread is wound tight around the spool. You can feel the tightness. Now slowly, pick at the loose end, let it draw out into the air. Once you have it, do not stop. Keep unspooling the thread. One circle after another, the thread will slip away. The tension will draw out with each pass."

The silence would normally be extremely uncomfortable at that point but—damn it, I kind of felt what he was saying. My throat felt *relaxed*. Or something. Now I don't know if he was really tapping into my chakra or if I was getting a contact high from the marijuana that had been embedded into every free surface of his palatial stoner pad, but I was starting to feel pretty good.

A sure sign I should leave.

I opened my eyes from the...trance? "Listen…"

"Van."

"Van. I have to go now. Keep an eye out for my dog?"

"Certainly."

I turned in the foyer. "How did you know my name?"

"Sometimes I bring your mail to you when it gets mixed up with mine."

"Hmm. And what is it you thought I had a problem with?"

He smiled. "Speaking. You're probably not good with

people. I assume you're the type of doctor that doesn't interact with patients much?"

"Anesthesiologist."

He raised one eyebrow and said, "It's all coming together."

I CALLED in sick on Monday and went to Farrah's. I didn't care that she didn't want to see me, I was going to get into that house. If she had died, I was going to be super pissed at her.

I-5 was rainy but it was midday on a weekday so traffic flew by as I passed under the evergreens of Deception Pass—a monstrously beautiful bridge that clung to rock clefts along Whidbey Island—metal archways spanning a devilish seariver torrent. I recalled a patient from a few years prior, a woman in her mid-seventies. Life had culminated in such a way for her that she decided to take a jump off the Pass. Only nothing about the fall ended her life—just gave her two broken femurs with no place to go. She lay there for two days, hypothermia creeping in like a poltergeist, settling into her bones. Someone found her and she was brought into us, body temperature of 82 degrees. Through colossal medical effort, she lived and left the hospital.

The only thing she learned from the experience was that she needed to jump from a higher ledge.

In medicine, Death is supposed to be the enemy. Death is the ultimate Sandman that lurks under every person's bed from the beginning of time. We don't like to talk about Him and we certainly don't want to look at Him, but He is there. He knows and waits for every single one of us. What started to confuse me is that we're supposed to fight Death like he is something to be vanquished. We're supposed to *fight* cancer and *battle* heart disease. But this war is uphill from the get go.

I started to realize that we had it all wrong—Death was no enemy.

Death was a sneeze.

A reflex. Death is just one big, bodily reflex that eventually comes to us all. Yes, you can exercise and eat right to maybe delay the Big Sneeze, but you'll feel that tingling in your nose at some time. Some people are better at others at stifling the sensation. Some people just...let it happen. Our error is the personification of Death—thinking we can outsmart a sneeze. But a sneeze doesn't think, doesn't plot—

Doesn't care.

I KNOCKED on Farrah's door with no answer. After waiting a moment, I pounded and yelled her name. There was a small scratching from the dog before the door opened up a crack.

"No visitors," the nurse said.

"Tell her it's Jude."

"She knows it's you."

"Tell her to eat shit and that I'm coming in there."

The nurse paused, trying to figure out what to do with me.

And then I heard Farrah scream. This was one of those blood-curdling, howling at the moon screams that makes birds flee from the trees. I felt the nurse let up on the door and I pushed it open. I leapt up the loft stairs and found her there, panting and sweating like someone had been flogging her with a barbed whip all night.

It was bad. Very bad. Much worse than when I'd seen her a week ago. She was skin and bones stretched taut over soiled bed sheets, convulsing and writhing in the crucible of cancer pain. For a moment I could only watch—there was something both terrifying and sacred about a person suffering. I wanted to yell at her for not calling me—not asking me for help. But I couldn't. I could only say her name, in a whisper.

I knelt at the bed and took her hand. "Where are your meds?"

With great effort, she swirled her head to me and gazed as if she were the reluctant demon annoyed that I was there to exorcise her. "Gone," she said.

"The pain meds are *gone*?" I fumbled through the empty pill bottles that had been tossed on the floor. There was nothing left. "How can they be gone? Didn't they prescribe you more?"

She shook her head. "Said I have to wait. Said they were giving me too much."

"Bullshit. Where is your oncologist?"

She sighed, exasperated at having to deal with me and her pain all at once.

I noticed the nurse behind me. I yelled at her. "You've been just watching her be like this? This is okay for you? You couldn't get her more pain meds?"

The nurse shrugged.

The same way I shrug after I couldn't save someone. I asked her, "Where is her oncologist's office?"

"Everett."

"What's the doctor's name?"

She told me and I left like lightning.

"I NEED to see Dr. Collins right now," I told the receptionist. I said it like a big asshole so she would have no doubts about me.

"Dr. Collins is seeing patients this morning."

"Well one of her patients is going through medieval-style

torture pain with her cancer on Whidbey Island at this very moment. She needs to write her a script right now for pain medication."

"Tell your friend to make an appointment and to come in."

"She can't get out of bed!"

My outrage had no impact—she'd dealt with the likes of me. "I'm sorry, but she either must come in for an appointment or be taken to the hospital by ambulance."

"That makes sense," I said as I steamrolled past reception and walked into the back rooms of the clinic. I noticed a woman in a whitecoat sitting at the back of the hallway and as I approached, saw her nametag. "Dr. Collins," I said, getting her attention. "Farrah Abdi needs you to write a new prescription for pain. Methadone and oxycontin. She needs it right now."

The woman stood, looking me up and down. "And you are...?"

"A friend of Farrah's. I'm also a physician."

By that time, the receptionist joined us with a security guard. "Sir," she said, "we're going to ask you to leave."

Ignoring the guard and the menacing way he placed his thumbs in his belt, I said to Dr. Collins, "Please. She's really suffering."

She shrugged.

I couldn't believe it.

"Have her make an appointment to come in. I can't be writing out random narcotic prescriptions to her friend."

"This isn't a *random* narcotic prescription. I know you've seen a thousand suffering cancer patients who need a thousand narcotic prescriptions. I get that this is just another work day for you—but it's not for her. She's...suffering over here."

She paused as if to speak, considering me a moment. For

a nanosecond I'd cracked through that hard exterior that doctors grow—shielding themselves from the human drama of their patients. And then the security guard grabbed my arm. "Sir."

I didn't feel like getting arrested so I left them there.

It's not often that I feel helpless. Farrah was only miles away, cancer eating at her bones and organs, suffering like it was the middle ages, and all I got were shrugging healthcare providers who couldn't have cared less.

An idea sprang up in the deep recesses of my mind which I quickly squashed.

"Bad idea," I said to the rain-soaked parking lot.

My phone buzzed. A text from Zella saying she loved me and that she found our dog. I put my phone away, rain drizzling on my head. Then I got in my car and drove to a pharmacy.

"Who is the provider, again?" the pharmacist asked.

"Um...me," I told her, clicking my fingertips on the counter.

"Oh..." she said, looking down at the prescription slip. "Usually the doctor will hand the prescription to the *patient* and they will pick up the medication."

"I know how it usually works."

Her gaze was on the prescription slip, eyes moving over the high dose opiates that I had scribbled there. She then studied me: saw my hoodie sweatshirt and dirty jeans that I wore when I wasn't working.

I shifted uneasily. "It's an unusual situation. It's a cancer patient in a tremendous amount of pain. She can't come into the clinic so I'm taking the meds to her at home."

"And you are...the doctor?"

"Yes."

"One moment." She disappeared into the labyrinthian walls of medications. I knew what she was doing. She was looking up my physician prescriber number, verifying that I was real and not some addict who had stolen a doctor's prescription pad. She was then googling my name to see if it matched my physician photo on my hospital's website. Likely she was also meticulously looking at my ID to make sure it wasn't a fake.

I wasn't technically doing anything wrong. However, if they knew I had a personal relationship with someone to whom I was prescribing opiates, the DEA might take interest in that little tidbit. They don't particularly like when doctors start setting up their own backdoor pill mills.

I wasn't exactly sweating bullets, but I wasn't the coolest cucumber as I waited fifteen minutes for pain pills that would have thousands of dollars of street value.

"Prescription for Abdi," someone said at a window.

I grabbed the white, paper bag and left without a word.

WHEN I FOUND HER, she had passed out. I checked for breathing and a pulse, and when I found it, I jostled her awake. Waking her up may have been the worst thing that had ever happened to her because she let out one of those horror-movie screams again.

I shoved the pills into her mouth. Delirious with pain, she fought me, but I got the pills down—enough to kill an elephant. But she was so tolerant at that point, it was all just a drop in the bucket of opium. Hours later, she came to. Her face was a withered prune—looked like she had aged fifteen years. Her hair was a rat's nest of gnarled knots, eyes injected with blood and her nose was a continuous faucet of mucous. As she drank from a cup of water, the liquid splashed everywhere. Every movement was a tremulous wreck. To top everything off, her sheets were full of diarrhea.

"Why haven't you been cleaning up after her?" I asked the nurse.

The woman had stayed downstairs. "Miss Abdi won't let me near. She gets violent."

"It's called psychosis. And it's from the pain. You still need to do your job."

I felt Farrah's hand on mine. "Don't," she said. "It's okay."

It was good to hear her voice—good to know that she was still there. "I'm sorry I wasn't here for you."

"Not your fault," she told me, her gaze meeting mine. Tears had glazed her eyes, creating an almost opalescent effect from the play of sunlight scattering in the room.

"Why didn't you let us visit?"

"It was only going to hurt you. To see me like this."

"But I could've helped."

"No. You couldn't. No one can—wait, why do I feel better?"

I cleared my throat. "I got you more meds."

Her face darkened. "How?"

"Doesn't matter."

"*How*?"

"I went to your oncologist."

"And she just *gave* you a prescription?"

I nodded.

But then she reached for the new pill bottles and saw the prescribing doctor: *Jude Rosen, MD*. The sound of the bottle hitting the wall from where she threw it startled me more than it should've. Her scowl was like some bird of prey, ready to tear me apart.

"I had to—"

"You fucking *idiot.*"

"You needed relief."

"You can't prescribe these types of opiates to an outpatient. Anesthesiologists don't do that. You'll immediately be flagged."

She was right. "It'll be fine—I'll just...explain."

She was gearing up to say more, to bring down hellfire all over me, but she was too tired. It worried me more than anything. Her anger was usually enough to power through the pain to berate me.

I told her I was sorry, that I couldn't just watch her in pain.

"You don't have to watch me at all. I don't want you here. I need a guard, not a nurse."

I ignored her and held her hand.

She squeezed it.

CHAPTER SIX

Once she got over her anger, we talked for hours—late into the night. She wouldn't say it, but I could tell she was happy I came. I knew why she didn't want me to come: to protect me. Ever since we'd broken up in college, she'd taken on a maternal role over me. Always watching, always protecting. Even then, on her deathbed, she wanted to protect me from grief. We ignored what was likely around the corner for her—ignored talking about the Big Sneeze—and actually laughed. Flashes of college and medical school cropped up. There was still fun—still life in her. And I wanted to squeeze out every last drop.

"Have you...thought about it?"

"*It*?" She was only playing dumb.

I waited.

"Of course I've thought about it. I think about dying every time I go to sleep."

"I thought you might want to talk about it at least once."

"What the hell is there to talk about? For all I know my existence stops with my last breath."

"You don't think there's anything after?"

"You *do*? You, of all people—the most pessimistic person I know—think you're going to heaven?"

"No—I just like the idea that you still might...hang around."

"Don't worry. If I'm still me—first thing I'll do is be your personal poltergeist."

"Good. I don't think I can do the rest of this alone without you pulling some levers for me."

I got home very late, Zella didn't question me—didn't complain. She knew where I was. She only hugged me as I kissed her forehead. The next morning, I couldn't stop thinking about Farrah. Alone and in pain. No relief. I wouldn't let it happen again. I didn't want her to be afraid of the pain. She would never suffer alone.

Never. Again.

I SHOWED up to work and looked at the surgery schedule. My name wasn't on it.

I found him in the hallway. "Lazlo."

He turned, waiting.

"I'm not on the board for a case today."

He studied me for a moment, a dumbfounded smirk on his face. "You didn't check your email over the weekend."

"No. Why?"

"Go check it. I'll see you at two."

I immediately saw it in my inbox under the heading *Disciplinary Action*. Of course, I'd entirely forgotten about Lazlo's spat with me the week before. He decided to keep me out of cases pending a disciplinary review committee over my "clinical actions". It was a classic asshole move that I really should've seen coming.

The meeting consisted of Lazlo who was flanked by Drs. Lafferty and Chikarus—two people with whom I didn't get along too well. Next to them were two others whose faces I barely recognized but with whom I'd worked with a handful of times. I did take a moment to reflect: since when did I become such a pariah? I barely knew these people, and those I did, weren't the biggest fans of mine. I guess ever since Farrah left the practice when she got sick, things kind of fell apart. She was one of those hardasses that everyone loved to work with: clinically strong with extremely good bedside manner. Everyone loved her. My association with her must've protected me. Now I was just a big, petulant child that couldn't play well with others.

I sighed silent relief when I saw Dr. Cappe walk in, the guy whose airway I saved in the ER. He *had* to be in my court. He actually gave me a small wave.

Lazlo started saying things and then I heard, "Do you know why we've called this meeting?"

I could play dumb or just get on with it. "Because of last week. When I left the patient in the recovery room to go to the surgical airway."

"Correct. This Clinician Competency Committee has seen fit to review your clinical judgement at this time and has temporarily suspended your attending privileges pending our decision."

I nodded.

The committee sat in rapt attention as Lazlo recounted the details of the incident. My colonoscopy patient had become too sedated in the recovery room. I was paged to come assess and was nowhere to be found. Then Dr. Lazlo himself arrived (thank the gods). He found the patient to be unarousable, with a pulse ox in the mid-seventies. In my absence, Lazlo decided to place the breathing tube as she was too unstable for any conservative measures. The patient was then sent to the ICU where she suffered from an aspiration event and was still mechanically ventilated (meaning fluid from her stomach went into her lungs when Lazlo put in the breathing tube). Lazlo then asked if I had anything to add to the incident.

What I wanted to do was stand up, walk over to Lazlo and point at *my* chair. He should've been sitting there and we should've been questioning *his* competency. There's something called a jaw thrust—I wondered if he had ever heard of it. I'm no zoo wrangler, but I could quite literally train a monkey to do it. When a patient is overly sedated, you place two hands behind the angle of the jaw and lift the mandible up, opening up the tissues of the back of the throat so they can breathe. That was all this lady ever needed. She would've awoken, and she would've gone home. Yet, Lazlo crashed into the recovery room like a cowboy, saw her oxygen level in the seventies, panicked and rammed a breathing tube down her throat. And now, she had gastric contents in her lungs and was still in the ICU.

But as I sat there a moment, thinking of my response, my stoner neighbor popped into my head. I thought about how he fiddled with my throat chakra—said I had problems speaking. Whether it was a coincidence or not—he wasn't wrong about me.

"My error was leaving the recovery area. I should have been available."

Lazlo tried chasing the shock from his face, but failed. His cheeks went red as he set his jaw. He thought he had me—that I would fight back and blame him. I suspected it was part of his plain to utterly dismantle my career in front of the committee and make a case to fire me. When he sighed and looked at the clock, I knew I had screwed up his entire scheme by admitting my own fault.

"Dr. Cappe," Lafferty said, "why don't you tell us what happened in the Emergency Department."

I couldn't have orchestrated the whole thing better myself. Cappe went over the impossible airway he faced in the ER—the enormous man in anaphylaxis. He spared no detail recounting how he had tried every instrument known to man to get a breathing tube from above. He said he had called for a surgical airway (usually done by the ENT surgeons) but that they hadn't arrived. He then sketched out to the committee how I expertly inserted a tracheostomy below the vocal cords and saved the man's life.

I may have shared a furtive smile with Lazlo.

"And, would you say Dr. Cappe, that the man would not have survived if not for Dr. Rosen's intervention?"

"Correct."

I went on to corroborate Cappe, that it was an extremely difficult airway requiring two anesthesiologists. I even added that I would make a formal apology to the ENT surgeons about being on their turf and taking the surgical airway from them.

There were nods all around.

Except for Lazlo.

They had me leave the room for a moment while they made a decision and brought me back. They deemed my competency sound except that I needed to improve working under the direction of whoever was in charge of running the OR schedules (almost always Lazlo). I told them I certainly would. They recommended that I take a couple weeks break from trauma duty and be placed in less intensive rooms at the direction of Dr. Lazlo. I told them that was certainly acceptable and gave a respectful nod to Lazlo.

After the meeting, Dr. Lafferty came up to me. “How is she doing?”

“Farrah?”

He nodded.

“Not well.”

“I understand you’ve been spending some time with her. Please, take the time you need to visit. We’ve let Lazlo know that you may need a few days off throughout the month.”

“That’s—thank you.”

And then I knew why they went so easy on me.

WHEN I GOT home that day, around noon, Zella was stressed with our little one, Kris—Regina was still at school. I told Zella I was sorry I was gone so often—that I wasn’t feeling myself and nothing was really making it better. Seems like as a physician I should’ve known that I was massively depressed, but—you know, we make the worst patients.

Zella was worried about her mom, a widow who lived alone in southern Washington. The woman had health issues with terrible insurance. We picked up most of her healthcare costs.

I told Zella to go to her mom’s, spend the night. That I would take care of everything. It was the least I could do. Afterall, I *was* a husband and a father. Relief flooded her face —Zella rarely needed help like that. She usually had everything so together. She said thank you in a heart-breaking formal way as if we’d agreed on some contract, and then she left.

When I picked Regina up from school, I saw her tiny scowl as I pulled up to the curb.

"What're *you* doing here?" she asked, suspicion in her voice.

"What does it look like? I'm picking you up from school."

"Where's mom?"

"Went to go visit your grandma."

"Oh. Is it okay if I just spend some time in my room when we get home?"

"Sure. What do you want to do?"

Her responses were overtly polite. "Homework. Video games."

"That would be fine," I said, realizing what I was.

I wasn't her dad.

I was her babysitter.

I HAD CALLED Farrah that night, asking her if she knew anything about a disciplinary committee formed against me and how everything magically went so well. She adamantly had no idea what I was talking about. She said she was otherwise doing okay with the meds I had brought her while once again berating me for being such an idiot and writing the prescription in the first place. She made me promise to never do it again and that her pain would be well under control. I knew she was otherwise lying—she would need more. The woman chewed through opiates faster than any patient I'd ever seen.

Without more opiates, another pain crisis was coming soon.

The next morning, I looked at the OR board and saw that I was put into a bunch of orthopedic surgeries: hip pinnings, tibial fractures, knee replacements. Fairly routine and boring but at least the orthopods were a fun group to hang out with. In the least, they put on good music—they were mostly metalheads.

I checked out a narc box from the pharmacy locker and locked it down to my cart in the operating room. I had a lot of patients that day so I drew up a lot of narcotics: midazolam, fentanyl and dilaudid. I placed them in the narc box and put a couple in my front pocket for my first patient.

Hello, they said. Hello.

I went and saw my first patient and was ready to get him drunk on some midazolam and take him back for a general anesthetic for a knee replacement. But the orthopedic surgeon cut me off, telling me he wanted a nerve block for him and for every patient that day. That surgeon usually didn't want nerve blocks but said he was changing things up. A nerve block is where an anesthesiologist uses an ultrasound machine to identify a tiny nerve inside a bunch of fat and muscle, and without damaging the nerve, places a needle and a catheter there to inject numbing medication. This can effectively numb an entire limb and completely take away any surgical pain. When you get a nerve block, you usually don't need a whole lot of opiates. The reason this mattered was that I had just drawn up about ten vials of narcotics for all of my patients that day who would no longer be needing them. So at the end of the day, I was going to have a bunch of unused opiates that would completely go to waste.

I did all the nerve blocks that day.

I also charted that I gave the patients opiates during the operation.

"GIVE ME YOUR ARM," I said to her.

Farrah looked up at me, confused. "What're you doing?" She was drenched with sweat, shaking. The pill bottles at the side of her bed were empty. Unbelievable. She had taken enough methadone and oxycontin in two days to kill Godzilla. And Mothra. Twice.

I put a tourniquet around her arm and started flicking a vein.

She tried to take her hand back but was too weak. "No."

I placed an IV in the vein, injected two milligrams of dilaudid and flushed it with saline.

"You can't do this," she said.

"Yes. I can." I was actually terrified.

When the opiate took effect, she'd become coherent and her wrath rained down on me like a meteor. All the work she'd done, she explained, everything she did over the years to protect me and my career—all to waste.

"They won't know—I won't get caught."

"You're using again."

A gave her a cold stare.

"Okay. You're not. How did you get it?"

I told her what had happened. I gave every patient a nerve block, so they didn't actually need opiates for pain control. I then charted in my record that, oh wait actually the nerve blocks didn't work that well and some of the patients ended up needing a little opiate. It really wasn't that uncommon of a thing to happen. Pharmacy would see that I had removed a certain amount from the narcotic box and reconcile it with what I had given according to the chart. Only all those opiates went right into my pocket, straight to Farrah.

She burned through her anger so fast that she could only

give me an exhausted glare. "This is the thanks I get? For helping you? You just put yourself in danger again."

"I never asked you to do all that. What did I ever do to deserve your help?"

She took my hand. "When you're family, you don't need to deserve it."

She was scarcely so cheesy. It was scary.

"Fine then. That's the same reason I brought these for you." I took eight more syringes from my bag—fentanyl and dilaudid—sat them on her night stand.

She could only give an exasperated gasp.

"I trust you can dose as needed, doctor."

CHAPTER SEVEN

I didn't feel like I did anything wrong.

I felt the complete opposite, actually. Yes, I'd diverted opiates, but they actually went to someone who needed them instead of the waste bin or a drug addict.

The more I thought about it, I didn't even care if what I did was wrong. What difference did it make? So a man takes some unneeded opiates—a cost of pennies to the hospital—and gave them to his sick friend.

I'd do it again.

THE NEXT DAY, she asked that I bring her more.

I looked at the phone a moment. "*More*?"

She must've gone through eight milligrams of dilaudid and one milligram of fentanyl. That was a lot, even for a tolerant cancer patient. After all the lecturing the day before, she was actually asking me to divert more. Why the sudden change of heart about me stealing from work?

"Is the pain that bad?"

"I'll need double what you brought me last night. Can you also bring IV methadone?"

"Double? Jeez—"

"It helped. A lot. I actually feel like myself."

"Okay, I think I can swing it. I'll work on the methadone, too."

So I showed up at work the next day and saw my name on the operating board: multi-level spinal fusion.

Perfect.

I walked by the pharmacy window, turning and scratching my ear as an excuse to glance in. No one looked at me expectantly—no one cared or suspected. It was just a bunch of boring pharmacists as usual. The method by which I had diverted two days prior was done in such a way that it wouldn't even give reason to think anything was missing. So I picked up my typical narcotic box—full of fentanyl and dilaudid—and made my way back to the pharmacy window.

"Can I get a ten milligram vial of methadone?"

The pharmacist looked at me. "Methadone?"

"Yeah. Doing a big multilevel spine fusion today. I want to front load the patient with a good kick of pain relief early on." It wasn't that outlandish of a request. While methadone does have the stigma of being associated with drug addicts, it's actually a hell of a pain reliever with a blood half-life of about thirty six hours so its pain relief lasts forever.

The pharmacist shrugged, said sure, and handed me the vial.

I worked the rest of the day doing two enormous back surgeries. It's an elegant little procedure where a neurosurgeon completely flays your backside open, exposing the vertebrae and then commences to chisel, hammer and tear the bone away, after which they try to put it all together in with dozens of screws running the length of the whole mess. Some people think this will fix your back problems. It's a deceptively bloody surgery as the back oozes blood for seven hours straight despite the surgeons stating there is no way they are having any blood loss. So I usually order blood products and lots of opiates.

For each case I charted that I gave ten milligrams of methadone each and then kept the vial in my pocket. I also did a little over-charting for the fentanyl and dilaudid and pocketed those as well. It's not like I left the patients high and dry when they woke up—I made sure they were loaded up with dilaudid and a nice ketamine drip. They were fine.

I left that day with thousands of street dollars in opiates. Just walked right out the door. That's the thing about being an anesthesiologist. People *expect* us to have narcotics on our person. It would be unusual not to.

Easiest thing in the world.

"HERE." I threw the ziploc bag of drugs at her.

She grabbed at it, inspecting the haul. "Didn't think you were actually going to get me all this. You're just charting that you gave it to the patient and then you're pocketing?"

I eyed her a moment. "Yeah..."

She was all business as she drew up a vial of dilaudid and flicked the bubbles out of the syringe with one eye shut, tongue sticking out. What she did next rocketed me so far off the planet, out of the atmosphere and past Jupiter that I actually gasped:

With needle in hand, she reached down to her foot and pulled off a sock. It was fast—a split second—but she knew she made a mistake.

She'd slipped into habit.

She played it off by itching her foot and then put the sock back on and proceeded to tie a tourniquet around her arm to inject into her hand. She acted like she was fumbling with the syringe—but I knew what those nimble hands were faking.

She had let her guard down for a second, and that was all it took.

I knew everything.

DURING RESIDENCY, I'd heard a story about an anesthesiologist somewhere in the Midwest.

This guy started diverting and abusing during residency, like me. But, unlike me, no one was onto him. He'd set up a daily system—managing to divert the opiates away from use on patients and directly into his veins. He had the foresight to realize that if anyone got onto him, they'd check his veins: arms but more particularly his feet. So he decided to try a different route of delivery to his body. Everyday, he got up, went to work and managed to divert a half liter bag of fentanyl from pharmacy. He custom made a sling around his shoulder, to fit under his scrubs, where the fentanyl bag could be placed snug in his armpit. He then ran a rubber hose from the fentanyl bag, under his scrubs and waistband, and directly into his anus. This way he could work all day and give himself a little squirt of fentanyl every time he squeezed his arm against his armpit. He managed this for ten years until he accidentally gave himself a concentrated dose and collapsed in the OR while doing anesthesia.

The point of the story is you can work—and work well—with industrial amounts of opiates running in your veins. And you can do it for years and years, with no one ever knowing.

Not even your best friend.

"How long?" I asked her.

She looked up at me, pausing.

It was all so obvious. The constant sweating, diarrhea despite massive doses of opiates, the runny nose—and why would she need so much methadone and oxycontin just to get a little pain control? That should've been plenty for any human body naive to opiates.

Tolerance.

"How long?" I asked her again.

I knew the look on her face—she was trying to figure out what to say. It was a rare look for her. She was a person who didn't hesitate to speak—always composed and knew exactly how to respond to anyone. Her wit usually had her miles ahead of anyone in conversation. But then, at that moment, she was trying to figure out whether to play dumb or just spill it.

She didn't try to insult me. "Long time," she said.

I had to sit.

I left her bedroom loft and somehow landed on a couch downstairs, my head actually spinning. I heard small creaks in the loft stairs from her footsteps. The fact that she even walked down the steps to me was an enormous gesture—she'd been nearly bed-bound for three weeks.

I spoke to her without turning. "After all the nagging—all the fear mongering that it could happen again to me—and you were doing it this whole time?"

"Yes," she said. The single word tore my world in two. The foundation of my entire sobriety had been built on the woman.

"So stupid...so stupid of me. This was why none of the cancer pain meds were working—they were just a drop in the bucket of how much you were already taking from work. Only you couldn't get them anymore so you were going into withdrawal."

"Yes," she said again, no less painful the second time.

I stood. She hadn't moved from behind me. I told her I needed to leave.

"To do what, Jude? To go inject? What does anything about my problem have to do with yours? It's been twelve years since you abused. My use has nothing to do with yours." I could tell she had that little platitude ready. It was her contingency speech in case I found out about her habit.

I didn't say anything else.

I walked straight out of the cabin—didn't look back, didn't look at her.

I still wonder what her face looked like as I left.

I DON'T EVEN REMEMBER the drive back home. I'd turn my mind into a blank room—four walls—with an ocean raging on the floor. Waves pummeled the walls, crashing against them, but going no further. That way I could bottle the chaos without it leaking out.

It was late when I got home, walking up my front staircase. I heard an owl hooting. I shrugged off the noise but heard the hoot again, realizing it was coming from my neighbor's front porch. I saw a figure sitting there, the embers of a cigarette casting a shadow.

"Dr. Rosen," he said.

"Oh yeah, the blueberry, chakra guy." I hadn't thought about him for a while. It was a miracle I remembered his name. Van.

"Getting in a little late?" he shouted across the yard.

I walked over—more for a much needed distraction than a neighborly visit. The reek of marijuana filled the air.

He scooted a lawn chair at me. "You don't look too good, friend."

I sat. "No. Not at all."

We shared an amicable silence and then I said, "That thing you did to me—to my throat chakra. It...kind of worked."

He grunted agreement but then said, "It's not your throat chakra I'm worried about. It's the heart chakra—that thing is bleeding black smoke."

"You're right, you know."

He reached his fingertips out to me, joint in hand. "Herb does nothing for healing, but it's a hell of a bandaid."

I looked at the burning joint. Usually when I was tempted, I imagined a stern look on Farrah's face from a bubble cloud above my head. But that was gone. Now it was replaced by Zella and the girls, sleeping just yards away from me.

"No," I told him, "I'm good."

My phone buzzed. It was a text from Farrah—a single word:

Sorry.

Might have been the first apology of her entire life.

"Mind if I sit here awhile, Van?"

"Saddle up."

I stayed up the whole night with him, talking about music and hiking. He kept offering his joint. I would've felt enormously justified in taking a drag and then asking for a drink. I wanted to flush twelve years of sobriety down the drain and be done with the constant tension and uncertainty about my own self-control. I know I've candy-coated my addiction into something that I just kicked out the door with the help of a good friend, but Farrah was right: the parasite never left me—it was only kept in check. Farrah, Zella, the girls, good job—all those things kept it at bay. Now that I knew Farrah was abusing the whole time—her entire career—well, it was like taking the wood blocks from beneath the tires of a Winnebago, perched on top of a hill.

But I knew, staring at that smoking joint, the only reason I wanted to do it:

Revenge.

Farrah had betrayed me and I would do it back to her.

But "No," I told him again, "I'm good."

I GOT home at 4 a.m. and heard Zella come into the bathroom while I was showering. I saw her figure standing behind the shower glass, opaque and pixelated like a censored image. I waited for her to say something—get mad, ask why I didn't come home—anything. But she walked away, silently closing the door.

I slammed two cups of coffee at work and then looked at the OR board. I was doing a couple back fusions again. I removed a narc box from the pharmacy lockers and found myself getting methadone again. Just because I was astronomically pissed at her, I wasn't going to let Farrah keep suffering alone in that damn cabin. So I did the cases, Lazlo looking at me through the OR doors every now and then. When I knew no one was watching, I pocketed the opiates and left for Whidbey Island right after work.

I texted Zella, told her I was going to see Farrah again. I promised myself that I would make everything up to her and the girls—things would improve. Farrah had no one and she needed me. Zella understood but I knew that it didn't make it any easier for her.

She texted back: *tell her we love her.*

It was dark when I pulled up to the cabin, the spit of drizzling rain in my face. The windows of the cabin were dark, a black pitch within. The hospice nurse would've gone home already. I opened the door and heard the dog whimpering for food.

"I'll take care of her," I said, opening a can of dog food. The dog took a full minute to piss outside by the water. I brought her back in and flipped on the lights. The searing anger I felt when I'd last left her had cooled, but I was still feeling like a demon ready to let my wrath spew all over her. I reviewed my opening arguments as I stomped up the loft stairs: *You're an asshole, how could you? You asshole, how could you lie to me this whole time? You're an asshole*—and so forth.

And then—

There she was.

I remember her face was darker than I'd ever known—a mask of ash and petrified wood—masquerading as Farrah. Her bed, the loft, the overhanging wood rafters—it had all turned sacrosanct. I was no longer in Farrah's room—I was in a temple.

I remember my knees hitting the floor.

I remember my breath going ragged.

I remember all my days turning trivial.

I didn't grab her hand—I already knew what it felt like. As I clung to the sheets, flinging them away, I thought I'd be flung with them—that I'd smash into a mountain peak or plunge into a lake somewhere.

Her cheeks were painted with streaks of salt. Her limbs had lost the laxity of the living—as stiff as a tree branch.

One arm was askew in bed, declaring its last deed.

Within the forearm the syringe still lay.

Hello, it said. Hello.

AND THEN I KNEW.

I knew why she had texted that she was sorry.

CHAPTER EIGHT

"Is Aunt Farrah still like...out there?" Regina asked from the back seat.

I wasn't entirely sure if I heard her. My mind existed only to catalogue and relay images of Farrah's body in that bed. Her face. Her arms—

No note.

She had no final words for me?

Wondering was the only thing that helped distract from the fact that she was gone. Was it the cancer pain? The loneliness? Was she mad at me? How could she do this to me?

I had never been more angry at her in all my life. The grief—the crying out and collapsing-at-the-moon, fist shaking, kind of grief—was the only partner to the anger I had for her. I thought her a coward. She couldn't make it to the end—it was too hard for her. And she could have at least called me after she had injected—I could've been by her side as she sank away. Anything...anything would've been better than dying alone in a dark cabin on an island somewhere.

"Dad?"

And she *tricked* me. Made me think she needed all those opiates—all that methadone—to help cover her pain and withdrawal. True, she needed them—but not all at once. She wanted them for one final purpose. The violation—knowing I was used to unwittingly kill her—was beyond infuriating.

"Jude."

"What?" I snapped, looking at Zella in the passenger side.

She swallowed. "Your daughter asked you a question."

I looked in the rear-view mirror and saw Regina, her brown eyes staring at me. Kris was in a car-seat next to her. "What is it?"

"Do you think she is still out there? Aunt Farrah?"

"She...she told me she'd be my personal poltergeist."

"What does that mean?"

I told her I didn't know how to answer that—that I didn't know how to answer any more of her questions. I wanted to tell her that I was so entirely emotionally unequipped to not answer her precocious questions or to even be her father. But I didn't quite go that far. I stopped at, "I don't know. Maybe she'll keep watch over me."

"Do you think she is still thinking about us?"

Zella took my hand. "Why don't we let your dad relax. It's a hard day."

"He's always Doomy Gloomy Daddy," Regina said, a bite in her tone.

Zella stared daggers at her.

SHE WAS CREMATED—A big eff you from Farrah to the world. There was a small service, including a bunch of people from work. Even some patients came out of the woodwork. After a few mournful nods and sympathetic furrows of the eyebrows, I was just about done with the whole thing. Lazlo had the audacity and arrogance to think any of us cared what he thought about Farrah, and got up and said a few words anyway. It would've been better had no one said anything. There weren't words to talk about her and the unjust steaming pile of life that she was served.

It was a perfunctory affair.

Dr. Cappe and Lafferty were there, offering condolences. "I'm so sorry, Jude. I know you were close. She really loved you," Lafferty explained, "cared about you a lot. She would've done just about anything for you."

People began to scatter once they realized how awkward and terrible it is to be at the funeral of a colleague who was your age. There was a woman hanging around at the back—she had a *look*. Cheeks hollowed to deep rivets—skin yellow like tallow. Her eyes were like burrowed scarabs: dark, shiny and writhing within the sunken sockets.

"How did you know Farrah?" It was less a question and more an accusation.

She looked me up and down, suspicion in her glare. "Friends."

"I was her best friend for twenty years. I've never seen you before."

"Doesn't mean we weren't friends." She turned, done with me.

I grabbed her arm. "What're you doing here?"

She ripped her arm from my grasp. "Hey man, I'm just here to pay respects."

"You can't get any more from her. No more fixes. Got it?"

True confusion flooded the woman's face. "The fuck you talkin' bout?"

"I—"

"I'm—" she lowered her voice, "I was her sponsor." She took advantage of the stunning effect this information had on me, and walked out. It was a tidal wave after the earthquake. Farrah couldn't have trusted me? *I* should've been her sponsor. *Me.* She was that proud? It made me realize all she did for me and all the nothing I did for her. She thought she was protecting me by keeping me from her addiction—always protecting me. Even her breast cancer diagnosis—I had to pry from her months after it was discovered. Every act was something to shield her good old boy Jude Rosen—

And then a sledge hammer of awful epiphany slammed my brain.

The overdose.

It wasn't about her—

It was about me.

She didn't want me to get caught diverting for her. So she cut out the source of the threat.

Herself.

I SLAMMED through an emergency exit and found a nice dumpster to lean on. It was finally time to sob uncontrollably.

I've never seen pigeons look at a person funny.

LATER, I was at home, playing board games with the girls. Zella thought it was a good idea to bring some normalcy into my life but it had never been so excruciating to be normal. After a few rounds, I excused myself and went to the kitchen.

I had an itch.

Zella didn't keep alcohol in the house—not even cooking wine. But I rummaged in the fridge—peeked through the cupboards anyway. Maybe there was some forgotten holiday gift of wine from a neighbor that wasn't thrown out. Rationalization is the lubricant of addiction: what is the thing that I'll justify to do in this moment, right now? I wouldn't actually go drive to a store for booze, but if there happened to be some laying around—hey, it's not my fault if I take a quick sip. I remember thinking that maybe I wasn't an alcoholic anymore—maybe I'd outgrown it and I could prove it with one, controlled drink.

But, of course there was nothing in the house. Zella was good. Probably as good at taking care of me as Farrah if I ever actually opened up and gave her a chance. I was about to return for another game of shoots and whatevers and then—

I remembered something—

Something beautifully awful.

I made some excuse and ran out to the garage and opened my car. My heart pumped way faster than any time I was actually trying to save a patient. I flipped up the seats, rolling them back, inspecting every crevice. And then I saw them, under a pile of socks in the back.

Hello! they said, Hello!

The last batch of opiates I'd stolen for Farrah: methadone, fentanyl and dilaudid. There they were, just sitting there. I traced my finger along their plastic vial caps. I waited, wondering if Farrah would posthumously stop me.

Farrah...

The garage was silent, moonlight streaking through the windows.

I took a few slow breaths, wondering about Farrah's legacy—about my girls, sitting just inside, waiting for their daddy. I remembered how it felt as the beat dropped in my heart, the opiate slowing its rate, slowing my thoughts. It was a plague to remember. I could just inject a little to take the sting out of Farrah's death—I knew it was a crutch but it could help me cope. One injection—and dump the rest and never go back again. It wasn't the worst plan in the world—

"Dad?"

Regina stood outside the car, watching me through the windows. I crinkled the baggy inside my palm. "What's up?"

"It's your turn."

"My turn?"

"In the game. Come on."

"Be right in."

I folded up the plastic bag, placed it inside my armpit and opened the garage door. After finding an overhang of the shingle at the side of the house, I placed the bag of fentanyl there—a small nook to hold my special secret. I knew why I put them there.

Just in case, the parasite said.

"Dr. Rosen." Van's voice from across our yards.

I found him on the porch, a pipe in hand. He asked me to join him, so I pulled up a chair. Though an odd fellow, he was at least astute enough to not offer me his marijuana again. He told me about all the messed up shit he saw about me in the stars or astral plane or whatever it was. None of it made any sense to me but just being next to someone who seemed to have at least something figured out was comforting in itself.

"Things are bad for me right now," I told him.

"Hmm."

I spilled a lot to him that night. Not everything. Not about the drugs or anything but about my job, Farrah, the girls. He listened like a friend. Not offering solutions, only an open ear. We played video games and drank soda like a couple of kids in junior high and then he said to me, "You're not leaving anything left for the darkness to eat from you, Dr. Rosen. You're doing its job."

His stoner platitudes didn't annoy me, I just drank the wisdom and went home. Late again, I fell asleep on the couch.

THE NEXT DAY at work was just another day. Just because it's your best friend who dies, there's still nothing that special about it. The only thing that was different about work was a plaque with Farrah's name and dates that she was alive. She smiled at me from the picture frame. I forgot how beautiful and healthy she had once been. I deeply wished that it was my photo plastered into that memorial plaque instead of hers.

Maybe it was a favor for feeling bad for me, but Lazlo put me back on trauma. I actually kind of felt like kissing the man —it was the only possible thing to distract me. My last moments with Farrah when she was alive were haunting me. She just stood behind me after I found out about her addiction, waiting for me to be understanding. But I left her there—didn't even say goodbye. I gave Lazlo a slight nod in the hallway which he returned. So we were basically besties.

A split second into my shift, a trauma code went off so I rushed down to the ER. I elbowed my way through the crowd and saw a portly patient on the table, struggling through labored breaths. His oxygen saturation wasn't too terrible—low nineties—on just a little oxygen in the nose. Besides his blood pressure being a little soft, the rest of the vitals looked pretty good. Before I turned to leave, annoyed that it really wasn't a code, I heard nurses whispering something that piqued my interest.

LVAD.

Left Ventricular Assist Device: when someone gets heart

failure so bad that they need a tiny machine pump implanted in their chest to help the blood flow. These devices do help heart failure patients live longer but they are fraught with problems and complications. If anything is even a little off with them, it's usually a sign of impending doom.

"Someone get an ultrasound in here," I yelled, forgetting about everything—forgetting about Farrah's wooden face, her hands, Regina asking if she was still out there somewhere. My mind was only in the present, dropping the baggage of the past. "Sir," I said to the patient, shaking his chest. His head lolled in some sort of attempt to answer. With blood pressure dipping, I knew he was starting to circle. Besides catastrophic vital signs, circling the drain has a look: erratic breathing, pale skin, a sweaty panic on their brow.

I heard the ER doc yell something to me over the crowd. "Pulse ox is dropping. You need to intubate!"

I ignored her as someone wheeled in an ultrasound machine and I squirted some jelly on the patient's chest. I ran the ultrasound probe over the chest, broadcasting a snowstorm of images on the screen. With slight movements of my wrist, I saw cardiac movement and honed in on the image: the heart muscle squeezing back and forth, the dark chambers within swelling and collapsing with each beat. But—

There was something wrong.

The walls of the heart were flailing—flattening when they should be squeezing, paradoxically emptying when they should be filling. As I explored more with the probe I saw it: the sac surrounding the heart, the pericardium, had filled with blood becoming a pressurized vice on the heart, preventing it from pumping properly.

"Someone needs to call cardiothoracic surgery," I told the room.

"We already have," the ER doc said, sidling beside me. "What you need to do is put in a breathing tube." She had an edge in her voice. We'd had a few run-ins before and I could tell she was sick of my shit.

"Bad idea. This guy has tamponade."

"Let the surgeons figure that out. Look at his oxygen sat. Put in the tube!"

I told her it was because the patient wasn't perfusing his tissues—that he was bleeding from the LVAD into the pericardium and it was acting like a noose around the heart. "We intubate him and it'll drop his blood pressure even more and right now, he needs everything he can get. If I put in a breathing tube, he's dead."

She looked at me like I was an idiot which was weird because I wasn't explaining rocket surgery to her.

"Fine," she said, "I'll put in the damn breathing tube myself." She turned to grab airway equipment but before she could do anything—

The patient lost his pulse.

"Where the hell are the surgeons?" I yelled, looking around to a bunch of frantic head shaking. "Someone bring a surgical tray." The ED doc was too distracted as she fumbled with a breathing tube to have heard me. Sometime during this, someone figured out that they needed to start chest compressions. Someone shoved the metal tray into my arms and I dumped the contents all over the patient's legs. I really only needed one thing:

A scalpel.

I felt along the bottom edge of the ribcage, toward the sternum, but I kept losing my bearings as the chest heaved up and down with compressions. After feeling just below the breast plate, I hesitated a moment—I hadn't exactly done this before.

But, I figured, the guy was dead anyway and I couldn't kill him *more*.

So I sank the scalpel into his chest.

Deep.

Everyone in the room looked at me for a moment like I had just murdered the man. The silver handle just stood stuck there, vertical in the air like I'd just planted a flag. Then I cut —hard and downward. I felt the fat tissue give way to the blade as trickles of blood oozed around my hand. Gingerly, I made small movements inward, waiting. Every millimeter felt like ten thousand miles as it sank in. Right when I was pretty sure the only good I had done him was put a hole directly in his heart, a geyser of blood erupted from his chest.

Perfect.

A liter spilled over my hands, pooling around the patient and soaking into the sheets. Another liter flooded over his belly as I called for blood products and saline to be given stat. His blood pressure immediately returned as the sac around the heart depressurized. As the circulation returned to his brain, he woke up enough to fight off the breathing tube.

The surgeons finally arrived, looking at me like I was an absolute lunatic. But, hey, I told them later, you can't argue with my results. After pumping the patient with bags of red blood cells and plasma, we crashed him down to surgery for a washout of the chest and exploration of the LVAD. We got him through it alive and breathing in the ICU.

Throughout the case, I didn't think once about Farrah. In an instant I had gone from the depths of sorrow to the clouds of possibility. In every other aspect of my life I was a helpless child who had no business being a father or husband. But put me in front of a dying patient and I felt only one thing: power.

It was a hell of a drug.

As I left work, I passed by Farrah's memorial plaque, the darkness easily creeping in once more. The high of the traumas had already burned off as I stepped out into the rain. Already, I was wishing for tomorrow, to be back in the ER—back into the fray where nothing in my life mattered.

In my jacket pocket, I squeezed around a fistful of fentanyl vials. If you had asked me in that moment why I took them even after Farrah's death, I wouldn't have known. I guess just feeling them in my hand was some sort of terrible coping tactic. They would be added to the stockpile I had underneath the shingles of my house.

As I crossed the street, I noticed a man in a suit looking past me. I looked over my shoulder and then back at him, his gaze meeting mine. Umbrella in hand, he started approaching me. I kept moving past him like I hadn't noticed the stranger trying to get my attention. I feigned fumbling with my keys as an excuse to not look at him, but he narrowed in on me.

"Excuse me?" he said.

"What?"

"Jude Rosen?"

"Yeah?"

He shoved an envelope at my chest. "You've been served. Cheers." He stepped off the curb and walked off.

I hefted the envelope in my hands.

It was thick and ominous with paper.

CHAPTER NINE

"In your career you'll get sued five times," a doctor in med school told us, "you'll lose twice."

Doctors get sued not infrequently—I'd been sued once before—and most of the time it isn't a big deal. I had malpractice insurance, that's what it was there for—it covered a percentage of the judgement if it didn't fall in my favor. I didn't open the envelope or call a lawyer for a few days. It was likely an anesthesia-related injury that the patient didn't know was a risk going in even though it was explained. Stuff like that was easy to squash. Or, I could've been named in another lawsuit with a surgeon in which harm was done by the surgeon and I was the attending anesthesiologist.

But when I showed up to look at the OR board a few days later, my name wasn't there. Soon after, my pager went off: please report to room whatever at some clandestine office high in the hospital.

The room was stuffed full of sweaty white people in suits —an ominous sign. It took me a minute to see Lazlo sitting in the corner, a beatific smile on his face—another bad sign. In front of the table of inquisition was a single folding chair. I stood at the side of the room until every eye stared at me.

Oh. The chair was for me. I sat, arms crossed.

A lawyer, dead center, started with the first jabs. "Dr. Rosen. I trust you've read the document that was served on you."

I looked at my nails and said, "Not yet."

There was some weakly veiled guffaws as the woman continued. "If you had read them, you would see the complaint brought against you." She waited for me to say something and continued when I didn't. "It's pretty serious, Dr. Rosen."

"Lay it on me."

"The complaint alleges medical malpractice against you and the hospital. There are three counts brought forward in the complaint. Count one is negligence through breach of duty to patient, causing harm. Count two is gross negligence by way of breach of standard of care. Count three is vicarious liability for which the hospital itself can be held liable for your actions."

The last part was why I knew they'd stuff a bunch or lawyers into a room to confront me about the lawsuit—their asses were on the line, too. "What is the complaint?"

"Negligence and gross negligence."

"No. Who has brought the lawsuit? What happened?"

"That, Dr. Rosen, is why we brought you here today. Do you recall your cases last month on the 12th?"

"Not off the top of my head."

"You were assigned as the physician covering the day surgery recovery unit."

"Okay."

"Can you please confirm that this is true?"

"Yes. I was the covering physician."

"A patient, Miss Roisch, had an uncomplicated colonoscopy in your care. After which she was safely brought to the recovery unit. Per the chart record, the patient had an oxygen saturation level of eighty five percent. The nurses then paged the covering physician, Dr. Rosen, for help in assessing the patient's airway."

Shit.

"Per the paging record, Dr. Rosen was paged three times without reply and without returning to the recovery unit. Is this true?"

"Is this an arraignment going on right now?"

"Dr. Rosen, we're only trying to establish the facts and create a timeline of the events. Now, is it true that you were paged but did not respond?"

"I was performing a surgical airway and therefore could not respond."

"But you were responsible to cover the recovery unit. Correct?"

I nodded.

"Dr. Lazlo was subsequently paged to come and assess the patient after which she was intubated for airway protection. The patient suffered a massive aspiration during the intubation necessitating intensive care. The patient subsequently developed acute respiratory distress syndrome, or ARDS, requiring ECMO cannulation—"

"She was put on *ECMO*?"

"Yes, Dr. Rosen."

SHIT.

ECMO (EXTRACORPOREAL MEMBRANE oxygenation) is a big deal. It's a life saving measure when someone's lungs, heart or both go into total failure. A patient is put on ECMO when the alternative is immediate death and we believe that whatever is killing them can be reversed once the patient is stabilized. When we put someone on ECMO, we shove big tubes in their veins, continuously drain the blood into an oxygenator and then pump it back into an artery back into the body. That way we keep the oxygen level high in their bloodstream while their lungs are recovering. The process of placing and maintaining ECMO is complicated and fraught with problems requiring highly trained ICU staff and a host of medical teams.

What I'm trying to say is that it's expensive.

It can cost around—

"—TWELVE THOUSAND DOLLARS, a daily cost to the patient. She was maintained on ECMO for a total of nineteen days. Adding in additional ICU costs, we calculate that the patient's total hospital stay is estimated around 1.3 million dollars."

"Are those the total damages claimed?" I asked.

She replied with an ominous "No" and said, "the patient is suing you, Dr. Lazlo and the hospital for hospital cost and emotional distress for 3.2 million dollars, all total damages."

I stood up and grabbed a fold up chair from the wall. While my audience watched in silence, I unfolded the chair, placed it next to mine and pointed at Lazlo. "I think you should be sitting up here."

The guy just looked at me.

The lawyer continued, "From what we understand, Dr. Lazlo is named in the suit only because his name was on the intubation note in the recovery unit."

"No," I said, "his name is on the suit because the entire

thing is his fault. The intubation, the aspiration, the ECMO—it was all because of his actions."

"Go ahead," she said, "explain."

"The patient did not need to be intubated. The only thing she needed was a little jaw thrust and some patience in waiting for her to wake up. The last thing she needed was to be put to sleep, have someone put a breathing tube down her trachea and cause a large volume aspiration of gastric contents going into her lungs. She got ARDS and needed ECMO, costing millions of dollars, all because Dr. Lazlo had poor clinical judgement."

The entire room still looked at me like I was an animal behind glass. No one was watching Lazlo for his reaction. There was something very...rehearsed about the whole thing—like they knew what my reaction was going to be. Lazlo gave me a tight frown but there was no worry in his face and then I knew. I knew that he had groomed the lawyers and the hospital to already be against me.

They interrogated me more about every detail of that day. They wanted to know if I'd had alcohol the night before or any other intoxicants. And then they asked if I'd had anything to drink the day of the complaint. They also brought up possible urine drug test (thank you Lazlo), saying that it was routine to get one in case it came up in court. They began coaching me on what I should say in case the media contacted me and how much I should divulge to my family.

"Settlement," I said, interrupting the automatons.

"What?"

"Why isn't the hospital settling?"

The lawyers shared a furtive glance. "We made a preliminary settlement offer out of court which was rejected by the patient."

"Then why don't you settle for more? If the record is so

clear, as you say, that there was a lack of physician coverage that led to negligence, then isn't it cheaper to settle for the full amount then go to court?"

"Dr. Rosen, why don't you just let us take care of those matters?"

"Why aren't you asking Lazlo any of these questions?"

"Dr. Rosen," the lawyer said, "were you or were you not the covering physician for the recovery unit and were you or were you not unavailable to help a patient who was in respiratory distress?"

"Hey, Lazlo," I said, ignoring her question, "how's the other patient doing? You know, the one I actually saved in the ER while you were killing this other lady? Huh? I think he's alive and well—not even in the hospital now. He would've died had I not left the recovery unit to perform a surgical airway."

He finally spoke, "That's not the question at hand, Dr. Rosen."

"Dr. Rosen," the lawyers voice rose, "Dr. Lazlo is also named in the complaint. His role and possible culpability will also be assessed."

"Are Dr. Lazlo and myself being considered under the same defense?"

"It has not been finalized if you two will be co-defendants. This is why we've brought you in today. To see if your interests align with those of the hospital."

"Of course they do."

"It still might be wise to also seek your own counsel."

"THEY'RE TRYING TO SCREW YOU," Gross said. He was a lawyer I'd used a few years prior to settle a lawsuit for me. He had this constant frenetic energy even when trying to sit still behind his desk—gesturing and working his jaw up and down. Neurotic and obsessive—exactly how I like my lawyers. He was expensive, but good.

"No shit," I told him.

"They're acting like they're on your side—that they're just trying to get a timeline—but they were really just assessing your personal culpability."

"But why? I'm a hospital employee. Wouldn't it be in their interest to defend me?"

"Not if they can blame the entire thing on your own negligence. If they distance themselves from you and paint you as a grossly incompetent and self-destructive entity, then they may be held less liable—and even sue you later. How's your standing relationship with administration?"

I hesitated.

"It would've been better if they liked you. You would think it would be in their interest to defend you but they already know they're going to be paying out so if they can paint you as incompetent or negligent, they may cut out some damages. Do they want to drug test you?"

I nodded.

"And?"

"And, what?"

"Will there be a problem with that?"

"No," I said, no attempt to hide my irritation.

"I'm going to be blunt about everything here that I need to know. In addition to the charting proof that you were not available during the patient's time of distress, the plaintiff will try character assassination on the stand. If they can get a jury to hate you—you're done. So forgive me if I'm blunt but it's a matter of millions of dollars. So, you're telling me there are no substance abuse problems? No? Or ever?"

"I said no."

"See, it's a response like that—all tense and pissed off—makes people think you're lying. Do better."

"There won't be any problems with a drug screen."

"Okay. How's family life? Any domestic abuse issues?"

I realized I hadn't even told Zella about the lawsuit yet. "I'm not home enough."

"The distant father thing. Yeah, I know that game." He shot a glance at a picture of his own kids on the desk. We both shared a moment of sheepish silence.

I asked, "So do I need to be worried?"

"Do I look like a person who worries a lot?"

I didn't know if he was joking or not. He seemed like the type of person who worried he had tuberculosis every time he sneezed.

"I get paid to worry. If I don't worry, people's lives get destroyed," he said. "I'll worry for you."

"What are you going to worry about for me?"

"I'll worry about," he lifted a hand and started enumerating, "defending you to the hospital. I'll worry about losing the case. I'll worry about punitive damages. I'll worry about your malpractice coverage paying out—"

"There could be a problem with that?"

He snorted. "Clearly you haven't had a big suit filed against you before. Some policies only cover a certain percentage of the payout."

"And mine?"

"You don't know off the top of your head?"

I shrugged, knowing I looked stupid.

"I got everything I need from you at the moment. I suggest

you get some piss to the hospital lawyers say 'yes, sir' and 'yes, ma'am,' and I'll get to work."

THAT NIGHT, I found Regina playing on a tablet. She didn't notice me standing there, watching her. Her pigtails swayed as she moved geometric shapes across the screen, fitting them into an ever changing layout of shapes and colors.

She turned and said, "Hey, dad."

She usually called me daddy. "Hey."

"There was a dead black widow in my room."

"What? Where?"

"In the corner. It's gone now."

"What happened to it?"

"It was there for a couple of days. It was already dead—must've starved. I could see it above my bed."

"Those are really dangerous spiders."

"I know."

"Well I'll go take care of it for you."

"You don't need to. It's gone."

"You should've told me about it. I would've gotten it out of there for you."

"A pack of wolf spiders came. They ate it."

"Oh."

She continued playing, never looking up.

I found Zella in our bedroom, she'd just gotten off the phone—face red and wet. Her mother was not doing well. The woman had uncontrolled diabetes her whole life—lost a quarter of her foot and half her vision. She'd lived in assisted living for the last four years, something we paid for mostly out of pocket—not cheap.

"Dialysis," Zella said.

"When?"

"Now. They took her to the hospital and started her on it already."

"Do they think she'll need it long term?"

Zella nodded, pain in her face. I knew there was more there than usual. She felt bad bringing up her mother to me—the costs and emotional burden. I could tell she felt even worse bringing it up in the wake of Farrah's death. As far as I was concerned, Zella's guilt was self-imposed—I never once felt bad about footing the bill for her mother. She didn't have anyone else and we weren't about to just let her rot and die somewhere.

"She'll need to get transferred to a new dialysis facility long term," I told her.

She nodded again.

I held her hand, grateful she didn't pull away—something she had the right to do. "We will take care of her. Don't worry."

I remember that embrace, warm and wet with tears. She shuddered in my arms. I was afraid the concern she held for others would balloon inside her and explode at some point. She internalized other's pain, bent and molded it to her soul until it became her own—she would've made a horrible doctor.

"You need to go see her," I told her.

She nodded. After she packed the bags and packed the kids, she kissed my cheek, said she loved me and left.

I remember wishing I could've explained more—tell her why I acted the way I did. Truth was, I'd forgotten why I had become the distant husband that I was. I had been mixed up in the fog of emotional war that I couldn't even remember myself—I'd forgotten who I was supposed to be.

I also forgot to tell her about the multi-million dollar lawsuit.

VAN HAD a party and his friends were weird.

I don't know why I went, but when I heard the music playing over the yard and considered the empty, lonely alternative of sitting at home for the weekend, I let myself in. Beautiful women lounged on couches while catered waiters brought hor d'oeuvres like it was some black-tie affair. A hookah the size of an upright piano had been set in the middle of the living room—an octopus god perched atop an altar while its disciples came to suck on its tentacle teets. Showers of fondu were found throughout the premises along with platters of a variety of illicit drugs—just sitting there for anyone. It was the worst place in the world for me to be. I felt like a character in a movie that you're screaming at to stop being so dumb.

I needed to leave.

I heard Van. "Dr. Rosen!"

"I was just coming to say hi."

"I'm glad you came, friend. You're always welcome here. Although you may not find these festivities your cup of tea—" His mouth screwed at an angle.

"What?"

"You are green with worry."

"I got a lot going on right now."

"It warms me to know I'm a person you come to, Dr. Rosen." The words out of his mouth were technically contrived but the guy had such sincere warmth, I couldn't help but be charmed by the man.

"I—" I noticed a man down the hallway. I ignore most strangers except for when they're staring right at me for an uncomfortable amount of time. He was dressed in orange flannel—thick rimmed glasses. His eyes were on me. Watching. Or was I just paranoid? "It's a nice party, but yeah, not my cup of tea."

"I certainly wouldn't want to...derail anything."

"Thanks," I said. I looked back but the orange flannel guy was gone. "I'll get going."

CHAPTER TEN

Brass tacks.

Anesthesiologists make good money.

Depending on where you live, you can rake in anything from two hundred and fifty thousand up to half a million dollars a year. This all sounds like a dream—how could a doctor have any trouble with money? Considering what actually goes into making a doctor, a physician's finances can get a bit complicated.

Let’s start with a typical, middle class kid heading out to medical school—a better start than most. He or she just graduated from college and, depending on where they went, might have some student loan debt. If you got into a medical school, you likely went to a good college, so you may have $100K of student loans if you weren’t a rich kid with parents to pay your way. Being a medical student is a full time job—there is no working. So in addition to tuition loans for medical school, a student might have to take out loans to live on for four years as well. This typically comes out to around $275K in additional student loans during medical school, all while your college loans go into forbearance and accrue interest because you have no money to make monthly payments.

So then you graduate medical school and start residency—which is salaried. But the pay is about $55K a year while you're a resident. Given our eighty hour work weeks, that comes out to about ten dollars an hour.

Yay.

Residencies vary in length, some are as little as three years some are as much as ten (if you're crazy and want to become a cardiothoracic surgeon or something). So you work for several years on a low salary, and if you live in an expensive city (like Seattle), you probably aren't starting to pay off any student loans. And—

They're still accruing interest.

In the meantime, your shitty resident salary isn't enough to even live on its own, so it's a fair bet that you're double dipping on your Visa just to keep your head above water—let's say to the tune of $20K during residency and medical school.

So you make it to your thirties and you're done with residency with no savings to speak of and you're around $450K in debt. All this while you watch all your friends who went into business and finance buy their status-symbol Teslas and bullshit McMansions. It's usually at this moment that you ask yourself: why did I become a doctor?

You remember when you get your first job and start seeing dollar signs. You're a year into practice and you tackle your credit card debt pretty easily but then the student loan repayment kicks in—at a minimum of $4K a month—basically a mortgage payment. And then you buy a home and get another mortgage payment on top of that. Then you have kids who sometimes need to eat and would someday like to go to a college (to insanely perpetuate the cycle you're currently in). And then your mother-in-law gets sick and needs to live in a high-end assisted living. All this while you're working one of the most stressful jobs on the planet. And then—

You get slapped with a multimillion dollar lawsuit.

A doctor's salary, although often high, comes at a price. There's no free lunch. It's a marvel that not every single anesthesiologist out there isn't getting high on their own supply just to feel a modicum of relaxation.

Given the mountain of debt and the general cost of even trying to live, I'd only managed to save up about half a million dollars during my 15 years of practice. Most anesthesiologists had much more under their belt but I generally felt pretty stable. It wasn't like me and Zella were big spenders either, our financial burden just was what it was.

However, I felt good with what I'd saved. It was of course much more of a buffer than the average American had so it's not like I was complaining. But when you look down and you're bleeding out and you see the lawyer sharks start to circle, you get a little worried.

THEY HAD FINALIZED the jury selection and were ready to start the circus. The hospital lawyers told me to not talk with anyone about the case, especially the press. They weren't overly enthused that I'd hired Gross as my counsel. The man was constantly in their business, asking for every memo and to be cc'd on every email. "It's my right as counsel!" he yelled at them over a conference call. "I must be given every scrap of paper that exists in your possession."

Fortunately, the hospital had decided to make me and Lazlo co-defendants rather than cutting me from their defense team altogether and casting all the blame on me. I'd initially wanted to skirt all responsibility to Lazlo, blame him for the whole fiasco. Gross explained that that defense would ultimately make me an adversary to the hospital. If the two opposing legal teams—the patient and the hospital—managed to convince a jury that I was fully responsible, I would end up eating the entire complaint and fees. So, I relented and found myself in the middle of a bunch of squabbling lawyers.

My father was a lawyer, and there was a reason I didn't follow in his footsteps: it all bored the hell out of me and I barely understood what was going on. Doctors know very little about law and lawyers know very little about medicine—combining the two would make for a hilarious 90s sitcom, but was not very funny in my actual life.

I didn't tell Zella about the lawsuit until a few days before the trial—I erroneously believed the news would burden her further in light of her mother's new dialysis. She was pissed. Not because of the suit, but because I didn't tell her right away. If there was anyone who didn't need protection from reality, it was Zella—she took extended release dosing of reality everyday and dealt with it like Ghandi.

I sat at the defense table with the team of lawyers, my reflection bouncing off of the glossy table. Did I really forget to shave for the biggest trial of my life? I looked over at the plaintiff—an emaciated women in her forties of whom I'd given anesthesia for approximately 45 minutes while a camera was pushed up her butt. Because of Lazlo, she spent weeks in an ICU and almost died. Sitting there, looking at my dumb reflection, I considered it the most absurd moment of my life—thus far, anyways.

When I noticed the acute absence of a certain asshole, I turned to one of the hospital lawyers, McQuay, and asked, "Where the hell is Lazlo?" She pointed behind us and I saw him sitting there. "Why is he sitting in the *audience*?"

"It's not called the audience."

"Whatever. Why isn't he in the penalty box with me?"

McQuay methodically cleared her throat like it was an imperative function before speaking and then said, "He was removed from the Complaint."

"*What*?"

"We met with the plaintiff late last night and were able to dismiss him as he had a diminished role in the incident."

"A *diminished* role? He's the one who caused the entire thing!" My voice rose, which was weird for me. I could be an asshole but I was usually the surly type with carefully controlled vocal intonations to deliver a metered dose of sarcasm. I rarely raised my voice and started to feel sheepish. When I saw that one of the jurors noticed my anger, I felt incredibly stupid. The judge then decided to do that runway walk thing they do where everyone stands up so McQuay took that as an excuse to stop talking to me, her alleged client. I looked over at my lawyer, Gross. His nostrils were flared so widely that I thought he was messing with me.

A booming voice cut the silence. "All rise for the honorable Judge Gutierrez." The enormous Judge lumbered up his steps and sat atop his pedestal, looking at me and the plaintiff like a referee about to decide the stalemate at a winner of a beach volleyball competition. Like a good judge, his face betrayed nothing—even that he was presiding in court. I suspected he wore the same, flat gaze when fishing or picking up his grandkids.

The plaintiff's attorney started with his opening arguments.

I don't remember much but it started with dire warnings about dangerous doctors infiltrating our healthcare system like some insidious disease. In a few broad strokes, he painted me as not only a blubbering, incompetent doctor, but one with nefarious and deliberate intentions to his poor client who got caught in the crosshairs during a routine colonoscopy. He stopped at mentioning my forked tongue and cloven feet. He went on to describe ECMO to the jurors—the life saving, heart pumping, lung beating magical box that costs a king's ransom everytime you pull the ripcord on the motor. With the drama of a soap opera, he crafted a narrative of the plaintiff's PTSD from her ICU experience and the untold years ahead of therapy and healing. He reassured the jury that he had stacks of evidence—troves of manilla envelopes and stockpiles of filing cabinets—all supporting everything he said about me and the case. It was all bullshit to the highest degree but that didn't mean the jurors weren't nodding along with his diatribe. He was good and he had clearly done this before.

McQuay got up for her opener, approaching the jury box. She rested her hand on the railing and emitted a measured sigh. She started off describing everything it takes to be a doctor—the training, the student loans, the long nights and sleep deprivation. She went on to describe the pressure and stress of an anesthesiologist—the critical thinking and situational awareness that is required to deliver safe anesthesia. I noticed the faces of the jurors immediately flaten. It's hard to get the average person to sympathize with a doctor. But McQuay continued laying the groundwork to then describe the reason why I wasn't there to assess the plaintiff—that I was assisting another anesthesiologist with a surgical airway. I was surprised to hear it—the defense team had decided to not include that detail last time we met. But, the hail mary worked as I watched the jurors open up to the fact that I saved the life of another patient while the plaintiff was aspirating gastric contents into her lungs when Lazlo rammed a breathing tube into her.

I knew the defense admitting I wasn't there was a gamble: would the jury care that I was saving another patient that had nothing to do with the case? On the other hand, the plaintiff had transcripts from the hospital records documenting that I was definitely not available for the patient, so there was really no reason to deny it in court.

McQuay recognized the terrible circumstances of the plaintiff's medical course but explained that it was a consequence of performing complex medicine in a large academic hospital. She bolstered this by stating that the plaintiff signed a consent form which included inherent risks and dangers of having a procedure requiring anesthesia. She asserted that being put on ECMO had nothing to do with the action or inaction of Dr. Jude Rosen. She was a pretty tightly wound person to begin with but I sensed an air of satisfaction with the way she cleared her throat and sat down.

I was feeling pretty good at that point. McQuay seemed to be on my side—was coming up with a good argument without denying the evidence that the plaintiff would show. For a moment, I thought things were going okay.

And then I looked over at Gross and his head almost exploded.

I KEPT WORKING.

I wasn't exactly chumming it up with everyone but I didn't cause trouble. I kept my head down and did my cases without arguing with the ER docs or surgeons. I missed Farrah more than ever—and not just as a friend but as a colleague. She would've had my back—would've coached me through the trial better than my lawyers. I touched her memorial plaque as I walked in like an elephant bowing down, remembering its dead.

I did a couple of urological cases which were pretty routine: scope up the penis into the bladder, putting stents in places that didn't drain urine. After my third case, I brought my patient recovering from anesthesia to the recovery room and turned to the nurse—

It was the same nurse who had paged me a thousand times to respond to the patient who now had me wrapped up in a lawsuit. I didn't know the nurse well, but I'm certain she did not have good things to say about me to the hospital lawyers and Lazlo. I suspected her puckered lips withheld untold judgement about me as a doctor.

I gave her my report of the patient, "This is a 58 year old with history of ureteral strictures—"

"Dr. Rosen," the nurse said, gesturing to a tiny man at her side, "this is one of my nursing students, Pete. He is shadowing me today. Will you give him the report so he can practice?"

I nodded and proceeded to give sign out to the nursing student. With wide eyes and rapt attention, he took notes about how the patient was doing and the medications that I prescribed for post-operative pain and nausea.

"So, what should I give for nausea?" he asked after I had just told him.

"Zofran."

He wrote it down and nodded. The nurse then told him to go grab a vial of the medication in case the patient woke up puking.

I turned my back and went to a computer to finish my

charting. It was about 4 minutes later that the recovery unit suddenly became very hushed. There are two bad signs that something is going wrong in a hospital: everybody talking quickly over each other or complete and total silence. Silence because some sort of error was made and no one wants to speak— they don't want to believe that whatever they did wrong is actually happening.

I looked over and saw the nursing student, Pete, with tears brimming his eyelids. "Dr. Rosen!" the nurse yelled, "we need you!" I walked over and saw my patient, completely blue. If you're wondering if medical TV dramas exaggerate what an oxygen-deprived patient looks like—they don't. The patient looked like Frosty the Snowman.

"I gave Zofran," the crying nursing student said, "that's all!"

I picked up the vial that he had used and—oh my sweet shit.

Rocuronium.

He made a drug-swap error.

Rocuronium is a potent neuromuscular blockade agent. Meaning, if I inject this drug into a patient's veins, it paralyzes all the muscles in their body, including their diaphragm—you know, the one that makes you breathe? I'll give rocuronium to a patient to paralyze their vocal cords so they don't fight as I put in a breathing tube. Their reflexes don't kick in when a surgeon puts a scalpel to their skin. I give rocuronium *after* I sedate a patient. Otherwise they have the acute sensation of being a quadriplegic person who can't breathe while evil doctors are doing things to their bodies.

So I was standing in front of a patient who was now wide awake and completely paralyzed from the accidental injection of rocuronium by a nursing student—blue as a smurf with oxygen level at 60%. It was another great lawsuit to hang my hat on and I was already wondering how Lazlo was going to pin it on me.

I yelled out two words: "Bag mask," followed by one other word: "Suggamadex!"

Someone put a ventilating bag fit with a mask in my hands as I stepped to the head of the bed. I gave the patient a swift jaw thrust and sealed the mask over the face as I started pumping. I felt air move and heard the pitch of the pulse ox start chirping up—although dangerously baritone. His heart rate in the 40s was also a huge sign that we were about to lose a pulse.

The nurse yelled, "The Suggamadex is here! How much should we give?"

"All of it."

"The entire vial?"

"Yes!"

She pushed the drug into the IV. At that moment, the suggamadex molecule was tumbling through his blood, finding the rocuronium and giving it a big hug. Suggamadex was like a sponge. It was chemically attracted to the paralyzing rocuronium and inactivated it once in contact. The beautiful thing about suggamadex is that it works in like 4.2 seconds—

The patient bolted upright, fighting me off his face, pitching the nurses from the gurney.

He took deep breaths, his pulse ox quickly normalizing to the 90s. I dropped the face mask and took a deep breath.

"Hey, Pete," I said, bringing the adorable nursing student by my side. The kid was trembling and gasping through his sobs. I asked him, "Guess who I'm going to ask next time to get me the right medication out?"

"Never me in a million years. It's over, I'm so sorry!"

"*You*," I told him.

He looked up at me, confused.

"Because now you learned to triple check the right medication every time for the rest of your life."

He nodded.

"Now you're a pro."

CHAPTER ELEVEN

"It's not good," Gross explained over his cluttered desk.

"I thought things were going okay."

He shook his head, eyes glued on mine. "The fact that they dismissed Lazlo is a huge sign—huge sign. The hospital is trying to minimize the damages, so the fact they bargained Lazlo off means they've made some sort of deal with the plaintiff."

"What kind of deal?"

"Well they got the total damages lowered to just under three million."

"Shit."

"Shit is right."

"So what do we do?"

"I think the defense strategy is sound—it's the best I could've come up with. We double down on the fact that you were doing your duty to another patient that was in more distress—an intervention which was life saving. We also need a good character witness. We must get the jury to like you."

"Who?"

He looked at me, bug-eyed. "You tell me?"

It was another of many moments where I knew Farrah would've saved my ass. I couldn't think of a single colleague who even knew me all that well. I was pretty certain no one liked me and with the sickness and passing of Farrah, I'd become a near social recluse that year. "I don't know."

Gross steepled his index fingers at his lips. "It's got to be someone sincere—the jury will smell bullshit if we put someone up there who doesn't really know you."

I shrugged. I'd been doing a lot of that lately.

"I'll ask around your department. There's got to be someone around that likes you, right?"

"...Right."

LATER AT WORK, I opened up an email from Gross and almost popped an aneurysm. It was a bill—

For seventeen thousand dollars.

I couldn't imagine that the man had possibly done enough work to be awarded the equivalent of a Volkswagen Golf like he had just won the plinko board on Price is Right. And I didn't have a clue how he already blew through the retainer I paid him. I looked at the itemized bill and learned why people go into law—they charge for literally everything they do. Every phone call, text message, call and response was listed. I had asked him a question in email a week prior and his one word response, "No", cost fifty dollars. I know, because it was on the invoice. Everything is billed in no less than 1/10th of an hour increments, so if the guy works exactly one minute, he charges for ten. I won't do the math, but one can imagine how quickly that adds up when he was charging $400 dollars an hour.

Usually when I know I'm getting financially screwed over like at the mechanic or airport, I pull out my credit card and move on with my life. But, given that I'd just dished out over ten grand for my sick mother-in-law, I wasn't happy. Gross of course explained everything over the phone with no opportunity for rebuttal or interjection. He made a compelling argument for the highway robbery. I did wonder a bit why he wasn't as passionate and convincing in the actual courtroom doing lawyer things for me.

He greeted me with a smile and a solid hand pump when I saw him again in court. I definitely hated him for more than a brief moment. McQuay sidled up beside me, not even a hello or good morning. Needless to say I had a dynamic defense team at my disposal, ready to dig in and fight for liberty and justice for Jude.

The plaintiff began their presentation of evidence. The plaintiff's attorney pulled down one of those old-school screens for teleprojecting—his face steeped in melodrama like he'd just unfurled the Dead Sea scrolls right in front of the jury. Slide after slide was projected on the screen, cataloging the events of the fateful day. He brought up the patient's charted vital signs—pointing with a red laser pointer at the moment that the oxygen level started to dip. He correlated this with a time-stamped page sent to Dr. Rosen and then showed three more unanswered pages. He then went on to catalogue the patient's lengthy ICU stay and how she'd developed worsening lung function after aspirating stomach contents eventually requiring the costly ECMO.

I watched the jury's faces as he wrapped everything up in a neat bow with an expert witness, some dickhead anesthesiologist from out-of-state who just parroted everything the prosecution wanted him to say: "Yes, I believe Dr. Rosen acted in negligent manner—yes ECMO is really expensive and could've been avoided for this patient if it weren't for Dr. Rosen," etcetera, etcetera.

I was about ready to call it a day until I forgot that we, the defense, had to do some cross examination and presentation of evidence, too. Gross questioned the expert witness, got nowhere and sat down. McQuay tackled the charting evidence, questioning the fidelity of how closely real-time events matched actual events in the electronic health record. The jury didn't seem to care. There was kind of a pause in my defense team as they looked at one another.

They sucked.

But then Gross said, "Character witness" and I saw Dr. Lafferty come up from the audience (which by this time had a fair amount of reporters) and sit in the witness box. Lafferty was the anesthesiologist who'd defended me in front of the disciplinary board—seemed to have some sort of soft spot for me because of Farrah. Turned out Gross did find someone at work who still kind of liked me. He asked Lafferty what I was doing while the plaintiff was getting a breathing tube in the recovery unit.

Lafferty stroked his white beard and said, "He was assisting another anesthesiologist with a critical patient in the emergency department."

I saw the jury perk up a little.

"And what was the situation there?"

Lafferty went on to explain that the man was dying—asphyxiating—because his airway had swollen from an anaphylactic reaction. With concise words, he recreated the scene: Dr. Cappe not having a clue what he was doing with the airway. Enter Dr. Rosen, who surgically placed a tracheostomy tube in under a minute.

Gross asked, “Would it be fair to say that Dr. Rosen saved the patient’s life?”

The plaintiff’s attorney stood. “Objection, your Honor. Leading the witness.”

Judge Gutierrez sustained the objection and so Gross reworded asking, “What do you believe would’ve happened without the presence of Dr. Rosen?”

“The patient would have died,” Lafferty said.

“And how would you characterize Dr. Rosen as an anesthesiologist?”

He leaned into the microphone and in the same tone as if ordering his morning coffee said, “He’s one of the best anesthesiologists I’ve ever seen.”

Huh.

For perhaps the first time in his life, Gross looked like his head wasn't going to pop. “Thank you, that’s all Dr. Lafferty.”

After Lafferty survived the cross examination unscathed, the jury looked less sure about Dr. Jude Rosen being such a deadbeat anesthesiologist.

A FEW DAYS later there was a knock on my door. It was Van, holding his phone up to me. It was a news article with my face. “Problems?”

It was the first time he’d come over to my house. “You could say that.” Zella hadn’t met him yet and I wasn’t crazy about her finding out that I’d been hanging with some stoner across the yard. But the girls were gone so I let him in.

“Wanted to offer my support,” he explained, “I can see your crown is dulled by worry. Your solar plexus is darkened, too. You’ve got too much on your plate, Dr. Rosen.”

I nodded and handed him a sparkling water. “I usually deal

with stress—compartmentalize it and work it out piecemeal. But now—work was stressful enough but then I had Farrah leave and now this lawsuit from hell. I'm not too confident about how it's going to go."

"What else?"

"Who says there is more?"

"Your body does."

"Zella's mom went on dialysis—we're paying for everything which is terrible timing. My lawyer is charging me a fortune and I'm having to work less because of the trial. Wouldn't be surprised if the hospital fires me after the trial, either."

"You're worried about money?"

"Of course."

Van looked around the house, studying it. "You do...okay? As an anesthesiologist?"

"Sure. If things were normal, I'd be fine."

He stood and moved to the window, looking out. "Is it your fault?"

"The lawsuit?"

"Yes."

"No."

"Then why are you worried?"

"Not sure if you've ever had to deal with lawyers and the court system, but truth pretty much takes a back seat to what you can prove or not."

"And is that justice?"

I knew he sounded like a college freshman who'd just walked out of his first day of philosophy class but I was listening. "No."

"You're a man who takes control of things, right? Takes control of the room, the patient, the sickness—you take control of your life?"

"Not lately."

He whipped around, looking at me over his glasses. "And why is that?"

"I—" It was everything. The safe guards had been taken away—Farrah, my job, my finances. The real Jude who I'd stowed away for fifteen years was emerging once more.

"Why do you let them do whatever they want with you?"

"Who?"

"*They*."

I remember trembling a bit. "I don't know."

He finally sat next to me in what was becoming a bizarre conversation yet not entirely unwelcome. "Do you think life is about choice or about fate?"

"That's the kind of question I would've asked myself when I was sixteen."

"And did you ever answer it?"

"...No."

"The answer is that it is both. Life is about *choosing* your fate."

"I don't know what you're getting at."

"You look out over the horizon of your life and you see hundreds—thousands of domino lines have been set up. Each domino sits upright, waiting for you to pick a line—waiting for you to make a choice. You pick a line and knock down a single domino. You've made your choice. And then you watch—as a spectator you witness the cascade of events that ensue from your single choice. You can't control where the domino line goes, you can only control the line that you pick."

"I get it. You make a choice but can't know the consequences that follow."

"I'm going to ask you one question but I don't want you to

answer it right now. In fact, you don't need to ever answer it if you don't want to. Because you're Dr. Jude Rosen and you make your own decisions—you pick your own domino line."

"What is the question?"

"After work, what do you do with the leftovers?"

ONE WEEK and tens of thousands of dollars later, closing statements were made. The plaintiff pretty much just copy and pasted their opening statements and pointed at me throughout the tirade. "You need to ask yourself," she pleaded, "did Dr. Rosen have a professional duty of care to the plaintiff and if he breached that duty, did it result in patient harm? That is the only question that you need to answer."

McQuay made an impassioned plea to not punish a doctor for having the medical acumen and triage competency to help a dying patient in the emergency department. "The medical world is fundamentally complex and with complexity comes risk. Dr. Rosen demonstrated sound judgement and acted in good faith given the difficult scenario in which he was placed. The plaintiff is not a victim of Dr. Rosen or the hospital, she is only a victim of the chaos and uncertainty that is inherent to medical care." Gross got up, basically gave the same closing argument and sat down.

The jury sat silent through the whole thing. I had absolutely no idea what they were thinking. I looked back into the audience and saw Zella sitting there. She was worried.

After the Judge gave some instructions to the jury—what the actual allegations were and whether the plaintiff had met its burden of proof—they evacuated in single file like school children and the door closed behind them.

An hour went by.

And then another.

AFTER FIVE HOURS OF DELIBERATIONS, the Judge released the court. Zella went home but I didn't go with her. I found myself driving to Whidbey Island. As I crossed Deception Pass—iron semicircles arching over turbid waters—my eyes fell on the churning water: inky black with a nimbus of moonlit fog. My mind revolved the same concepts: sunset, death, birth, killer. Raw philosophy emerged: *There is no day without night. There is no health without disease. There is no gain without robbing.* My job had already dragged me into the throes of fatalism, but then, in that moonlight, while my life was being determined by twelve people who didn't know me—deep nihilism set in.

What I did didn't matter.

I opened the door to Farrah's cabin.

I didn't turn on the lights.

The place smelled of disinfectants and cardboard.

I sat in the darkness, and, unbeknownst to me, a little gnome in the back of my brain was tabulating choices, analyzing risk and estimating probabilities. The gnome crunched the numbers over and over again but kept coming to the same conclusions.

Conclusions that were obvious in retrospect. Decisions that were formed long before my executive functions considered them. Looking back, it's easy to see what I was going to do. But when you're in the moment, you build mental walls of deniability and rationalizations. You keep your multi-faceted morals facing outward, to neither reflect upon nor consider one another.

Isolation is key.

I AWOKE the next morning to my phone buzzing—a text from Gross telling me to get my ass to court.

The jury had made a decision.

My back ached from where I'd slept in a sofa chair all night. I looked around the cabin one last time, watching motes of dust fall in sunbeams between the overhead rafters. The place was a tomb and brought me no solace. I was surprised it hadn't been sold off yet. And what had happened to Farrah's dog? It was the first time I realized I should've stuck around to help with her affairs. I added it to the list of things I did poorly.

After cinching my tie, I opened the double doors to the courtroom and saw the entire host of the court look back at me. McQuay snorted derisively as I sat—Gross just shook his head. I didn't know what the big deal was. The jury had already made a decision, it's not like my tardiness was suddenly going to tip the scales.

What proceeded was very much like what you see in movies. One juror, beckoned by the Judge, came forward, envelope in hand. A tense silence enveloped the room while the Judge read the verdict to himself. He handed the papers back and gestured for the juror to speak. It was a small-framed woman, her wide eyes exposing anxiety.

"On count one, negligence and breach of duty to cause harm, we the jury find Jude Rosen guilty. On count two, gross negligence and breach of standard of care, we the jury find the defendant not guilty. On count three, vicarious liability, we find the defendant guilty."

I thought two out of three wasn't too bad but I looked at Gross—he wouldn't look at me. McQuay—she was already packing up her briefcase.

The Judge took over the show. "In review of the verdict of this jury, the court deems fit to order the jury's recommendation of full payment of 2.8 million dollars, awarded to the plaintiff. This does not include the payment for the plaintiff's attorney fees, of which this court finds the defendant responsible."

Then he hit his gavel on the thing.

Then the show was over.

But the credits didn't roll.

CHAPTER TWELVE

I woke up to a phone call from an unknown number. "Is this Jude Rosen?"

"Yeah?"

"Dr. Rosen, my name is Judy Cliver, attorney at—"

"I don't need any more lawyers."

"Well, you see—"

"Stop. I don't want to hear it."

"Dr. Rosen, if you'll let me explain—"

Click.

I'd had more than enough legal counsel for a lifetime—which cost about a lifetime of salary. I'd gotten my final bill from Gross.

It was only the beginning.

The hospital's malpractice insurance did pay for the bulk of the lawsuit payout, my insurance paid the rest. If not for the insurance, I would've been bankrupt immediately. I was also held responsible for the plaintiff's legal fees. It totaled somewhere over one hundred thousand. So as I was hemorrhaging cash through my savings account, the patient decided to go for the gold and slap me with punitive damages. Punitive damages are reserved specifically for people that you want to punish—someone that has screwed you over so badly that you want to drain them of every last penny to their name.

My personal judgement and legal fees were over four hundred thousand dollars. I refused to claim bankruptcy.

"WHAT'S LEFT OF SAVINGS?" Zella asked, eyes focused on the sheets of invoices, pay stubs and bills that I'd brought out over the kitchen table. It represented the current ins and outs of our finances. Her mom's hospital bills were well represented.

"I just drained the last of it."

"*All*?"

I nodded.

As I stood there looking at my wife, hearing my children play in another room, I wanted to be alone in a room with Lazlo. Just me and him. I wasn't a vindictive person—usually too lazy to muster the energy required to hate someone. But Lazlo had pushed me. His one stupid idea to put a breathing tube in a patient cost me everything—I had no savings for my girls.

Zella was suddenly at my side, her hand in mine. "It's okay."

I told her, "No. It's not," and let go, her optimism only irritating me.

"We'll find a way."

"Sometimes there isn't anything positive in a situation, Zella." It was weird that I said her name, I rarely actually called her that.

"You're still bringing in a lot of income—"

"If I still have a job."

"...And we can start our savings back up again—"

"If the medical board doesn't revoke my license."

"They would do that?"

I shrugged. "My case will be under review. If they think I'm as reckless of a doctor as the court, they could take my license away."

"I don't think that will happen—"

"And we haven't even paid everything off yet. I've no idea where we're going to come up with the money."

"We'll figure it out—"

"Just stop," I told her, "sometimes things don't work out. You know that, right?"

She was done with me, walked out of the room.

I wanted to be done with me, too.

I SHOWED up at work that Monday and was listed to start a case in the OR. Somehow I still had a job. I wasn't sure what I was going to do when I saw Lazlo. I was afraid it would end in my arrest and imprisonment thereafter.

So I avoided everyone as much as I could and prepared for my first case. I unlocked my narcotic box, the memory of Farrah with a needle in her arm flitted across my mind. I shuddered for a moment, the itch of impotence creeping through me —sapping me of the will to even put one foot ahead of another. I hadn't even processed the death—the suicide—of my best friend and I was suddenly financially demolished in little over a month. It was a miracle I wasn't diverting opiates directly up my own ass at that point. Maybe I had changed—maybe the parasite was gone.

I did the anesthesia for a plastic surgery case. For five hours I watched as the surgeon grafted skin from a shoulder into the skin of the neck from a prior burn injury. I normally would've been bored, but the lack of action only allowed the depression to soak into my brain.

I pocketed a couple vials of fentanyl—why not? I wasn't sure what I was going to do with them. But I kind of was.

"Jude," a voice called from the door. It was Lafferty. He came in and put his hand on my shoulder. "How's the day going?"

"Going better knowing that I still have a job."

His eyes squinted above the surgical mask. "I'm sorry that it was in question."

"I should be fired."

"Why?"

"I cost the hospital millions of dollars."

"True."

"So?"

"It was a big lawsuit, I'll admit. But we build in a financial cushion for such lawsuits. They happen—they'll happen again. You were just the poor bastard who happened to be involved. Your defense team was right, that woman was a victim of circumstance, not a victim of Jude Rosen."

"You're telling me Lazlo hasn't tried to get me fired?"

He tilted his head. "Dr. Lazlo isn't the final word around here. Have you ever thought that you're not fired because you're actually good at what you do?"

"I—"

"And that you've prevented more patient deaths than anyone I've ever seen?"

"I...thank you."

"Don't thank me. Just keep doing what you're doing. And when you're done here, go look at the OR board."

I finished my case and found out what I was doing next: a liver transplant.

For the next twelve hours, I was elbow deep in blood products: pumping dozens and dozens of blood cells, platelets, plasma and cryoprecipitate into a liver cirrhotic who was continuously trying to die on the table. I was like the pilot in a plane going down—constantly pulling levers, slamming buttons and pushing medications. I floated a balloon catheter into the patient's heart to get more sensitive readings of the patient's specific cardiac chambers.

Everything else just slipped away.

My heart pumped with the knowledge that every decision—every flick of my wrist—would save or kill the patient.

The surgeon managed to get the new liver in, stapled up and with the bleeding controlled. I dropped the patient in the ICU, bloated and oozy—but alive.

The demons had receded—the thrill of the OR keeping them at bay.

THAT WEEKEND I checked my bank account.

I hadn't been paid.

After a few long and confusing conversations with billing and payroll, the explanation was quite simple: my wages were being garnished.

"So...how do I stop it?"

"You don't," they explained, "that's what garnishing is. Once you stop paying money to people that you owe, they just take it directly out of your paycheck. You can't stop it."

After I hung up the phone, I did some quick math, adding up everything I still owed divided by how often I got paid. I shuddered as I looked at the calculator. At the rate they were stealing my money, I wouldn't have the damages paid off for another eighteen years—

Eighteen. Years.

AFTER A FEW ANGRY PHONE CALLS, I did manage to funnel some of my own paycheck back to me and my adorable attempt to provide for a wife and two children. As I broke down the numbers, it wasn't enough to sustain the mortgage and our current lifestyle. We were going to have to pull Regina out of the fancy charter school, too.

"Can we move? Can you get a job in another state?" Zella asked.

"They'll find me. And that's given I can even get hired at another job. I'd have to disclose the malpractice suit and then no one will touch me."

"We have equity in the home."

I shook my head. "No bank would give me a loan to buy another house."

"We'll move to a cheaper part of town. We'll rent while we save up again."

"What about your mom?"

Zella's face went white. "I'll get a job. I can go back to nursing. I *have* to."

I nodded. "Okay," I said to her, more trying to console myself. "Maybe we can get it to work."

ZELLA TOOK a job back at my hospital. It was painful hiring a nanny with everything so tight, but it made financial sense in the end. Regina hated the woman—hated Zella for allowing it to happen—and hated me for basically everything else.

So we limped on for another couple of months, opting to defer mortgage payments for a month or two while our new shit show finances stabilized. The bulk of our income was going to Zella's mom, who was doing quite fine given she was getting her dialysis every other day.

Throughout the great depression of the Rosen family, I found my mind wandering back to that night I spent in Farrah's cabin, alone, while a jury decided my fate. That night, the moon or the fog brought some sort of clairvoyant clarity to my life. I could see the different possibilities—the various domino lines, as Van would put it. I knew what my life would look like if I were found guilty, and all of it had come to fruition. I'd be consigned for the next several years paying a debt to someone who I didn't harm—a patient who was now profiting off my daily labor.

I thought of Lazlo.

A lot.

Sometimes we'd connect eyes for a moment in the hallway. He'd feign distraction and walk the opposite direction. I was relieved to watch him walk away from me. I never got in a conversation with him once since the trial—I was too afraid. After I had a dream involving a piano wire and his neck, I was genuinely afraid I wouldn't be able to stop myself from hurting the man. More haunting was the fact that I knew where he lived—knew his work schedule—I knew exactly where he parked everyday. If I wanted to, I could get revenge in a very serious way.

I'd been many unsavory things in my life—including an addict and alcoholic—but I'd never descended to violence. I was becoming some sort of shriveled up goblin living under a dank bridge, muttering to myself about all the people that had wronged me and the numerous ways in which they'd pay.

Including Lazlo.

I watched people die everyday—there was nothing special about it. I'd give 2 ccs of a medication to save a life—I could just as easily give 2 ccs of a different medication to take a life. Did it matter? These thoughts are usually absurd and short lived, but when fueled by what I could only think of as righteous indignation—these thoughts turn to impulse incredibly easy. I was finally starting to understand those bizarre news headlines about people shooting up their work place or setting their own homes on fire with their loved one still there—

When you find yourself sympathizing with the unhinged of society—you're in a pretty dark place.

I was terrified of what I was becoming and that stern look that Farrah was giving me from a bubble cloud above my head was quickly evaporating.

IT WAS 5am on a Monday morning.

I was sitting in my car. A blood red dawn had spilled into the horizon and the low lighting of the parking garage offered the visibility of a rock concert. In the stillness of the early morning, I waited. I waited another ten minutes. I don't remember taking a breath.

The silver Mercedes pulled in and parked.

My fists clenched.

I wasn't me. Someone else—something else had taken the cockpit.

It was all those nights—pumping on people's chests. It didn't matter. Death was just a blink of the eyes—the Big Sneeze that comes for everyone. This was the prevailing mantra and it was currently working.

Lazlo got out of his car, lifting a bag to his shoulder.

I got out of my car.

He shut the car door, heading for the hospital doors. I matched his pace, my footsteps silent.

He didn't notice a clatter at his feet as he opened the doors.

I was right behind him—the garage empty.

"Lazlo," I said, almost a whisper.

When he saw me standing there, fear swept his face.

A century of silence lasted between us as I stared at him. Finally, I walked up and reached at his feet.

"You dropped your pen," I said, offering it back.

He swallowed and then took it. "Thank you," he said before quickly entering the hospital.

"You're welcome," I said to no one.

"DR. ROSEN," Van said, a smile lifting on his face. He stood in the doorway, drinking in my sudden appearance at his home. "It is *so nice* to see you."

I lifted a brown paper sack to him.

He stared at it a moment and said, "Are you sure?"

"I'm about to become something much worse if you don't take this."

He took the bag and, after opening it, a tiny gasp escaped his lips.

CHAPTER THIRTEEN

I told myself I had no other options.

It was either relieve me and my family of our financial purgatory or go supernova.

That was it.

I still wonder what would've happened if I had more than just my fists that morning in the parking garage with Lazlo.

It was the hate that got under my skin—like a small infection getting into a scratch. I didn't notice the cut—the small line of inflammation on the back of my calf. But it festered, turning into an abscess of resentment and then disseminating to the bloodstream, seeding to the rest of the body. It's when the hate gets to the mind that you can no longer ignore it. The problem is, once the hate is in the brain, you can't think straight. Like a virus, it starts driving your heart and mind toward the only cure: revenge.

Liquid hot revenge. But being a novice at the whole vengeance thing, I was pretty sure I was on the verge of destroying my life more than it had already been.

So I came up with a loophole.

"No phone calls, no texts—ever again," Van said.

I nodded.

"In fact, remove my number from your phone entirely. You never call me—not even on a burner."

I nodded again and whipped out my phone. I knew what Van was—I knew the whole time.

"When you've got something for me, you knock on my back porch window. If I'm not there, come back another time. We won't be making appointments." He was a different person—the airy tone of mysticism had left his voice as he explained his business operations inside his mansion bought with drug money.

My palms were sweaty. True, I was desperate for cash and a way out of the dank hole of bitterness I'd dug, but I was nervous. Van undoubtedly had guns somewhere and knew how to use them. I'd never even seen a gun in real life except on the belt of a cop. I had no idea what I was doing but it was already providing excellent sublimation from the thoughts of wanting to attack a co-worker.

"Anything else?" I asked him.

He leaned in close, the leather couch squeaking beneath him. "Can you bring more fentanyl?"

I nodded.

"As much as the bag you brought me?"

I nodded again. "More." I felt better saying as few words as possible.

"Wait here." He got up, leaving me alone in the cavernous basement full of arcade games and other stupid things people his age enjoyed. I wondered how he was able to flaunt so much cash around without the IRS getting at least a little curious. He was either very smart or very dumb. Probably both. I wondered if he worked alone or was partnered with someone else—some sort of multi-level marketing for drug lords.

He came back in the room and threw a paper bag in my lap. When I put my hand in, I didn't expect to feel an actual *stack*. I flipped through the bills.

It was seven thousand dollars.

I tried to hide my surprise. I hadn't even given him that many opiates. Maybe ten vials of fentanyl, twelve of dilaudid and a couple methadone—the leftovers. I could collect the same amount in just a few days of working in the ORs. Probably more. "Good," I said.

He lifted his face, studying me. "And, we should probably...cease our social pleasantries."

"Agreed." I stood and moved to the sliding door. "Van…"

He looked at me.

"What do you see?" I asked him.

"Hmm?"

"In my auras or chakras or whatever?"

He studied me for a moment and then said, "Nothing. There's nothing there."

I SAW Zella washing her face in the bathroom. "Hey," I said, putting my hand on her back.

"I gotta get up early tomorrow."

"I'm going to pick up some moonlighting shifts. We should be able to start paying the mortgage again."

"Won't they just garnish it?"

"It's at a hospital down in Federal Way. I should be able to at least get a few months of paychecks before they figure it out."

"That's great," she said in a tone suggesting she didn't think it was great. Her voice was small, squeaky and distant. We'd mostly been communicating in head nodding and gestures.

"We can keep some savings for your mom, too," I told her.

She nodded and continued scrubbing in the mirror.

I visited Kris and Regina in their bedrooms and pulled a book off the shelf. "Story time?" I asked them. Kris' face lit up but Regina shook her head.

"I've already read that one," Regina said like a little brat.

"You don't want to hear it again?"

"No. I already know it." She turned her back to me. I went to leave but then heard her ask, "Are you and mom going to get a divorce?"

Divorce?

Had things gotten that bad?

My mistake was a microsecond of hesitancy—children are experts at reading responses to close ended questions. "Of course not," I said.

"I don't believe you," she said, never having turned to face me.

I stood there a moment, a child's book falling from me fingers. I knew what I had been turning into those last few months—a classic bad dad. The distant, workaholic, stressed-out-of-his-mind type of dad. But while I watched Regina fake that she was falling asleep in front of me, I knew I'd become something new. The one exchange between Van earlier that day had rocketed me into higher echelons of bad dads.

I was tabloid worthy.

THE NEXT MORNING, I'd use the seven grand to pay off the rest that I owed to Gross (he kindly reminded me that after doing some auditing, he'd undercharged me for his excellent services). So, knowing that I had no savings and was indebted to pay off the lawsuit debt for the next several years, I got to work.

"Can you put me in a spine room tomorrow?" I asked Lazlo. It was our first interaction since the parking garage. I didn't know just how much it startled him until I saw his response. There were no furrowed eyebrows or pregnant pause as if addressing a child.

"No problem," he said before going to the computer to change the OR assignment.

The next day I went to the pharmacy window. "Doing a bunch of spines again today—three," I told the pharmacist. "I want a bag of fentanyl infusion for each case."

"A *bag*?"

"Yes. 500 ccs. I'm going to do a fentanyl infusion for each patient. The lipophilicity of fentanyl gives it a nice duration of action—it'll help with post-operative pain by having an infusion going for a couple of hours." I found that using big, doctor-words helped people not question what you wanted.

"We don't usually do fentanyl infusions."

"I'd like to try it. I'm thinking of doing a study to compare a fentanyl infusion to our standard dilaudid and methadone."

"Okay..." she said, bringing up a clipboard. "Sign here and we'll have them delivered to your OR."

I also checked out a narcotic lock box with vials of fentanyl and dilaudid. Once I was in the first spine case, I sent the patient off to sleep, put a breathing tube in and flipped her onto her stomach. While the surgeons slapped iodine on the back and prepared to cut, a pharmacy tech brought the bag of fentanyl. I held it in my hands for a moment, distracted by the ambient light scattering through the clear liquid.

Once the surgeons started the operation and the scrub and circulator nurses were distracted, I grabbed a 500cc bag of normal saline—identical in appearance to which the fentanyl bag was prepared. I tore the fentanyl label off of the genuine article, slapped it on the dummy bag and started infusing it into the patient. I slipped the bag of fentanyl into my scrub jacket pocket and, when Dr. Cappe came to give me a break, ran up to my locker and placed the bag of fentanyl there.

"Fentanyl infusion, huh?" Cappe said, pointing to the dummy bag when I came back.

"Yeah. I've been having issues with uncontrolled pain in these cases lately, thought I'd try this."

He shrugged. "Not a bad idea. Better make sure you turn it off in time or that patient won't be waking up for a *long* time."

"Of course."

Once the surgery ended, I woke up the patient and took out the breathing tube. The entire room scowled at me as the patient howled in pain. Quickly, I worked in a bunch of dilaudid until she fell asleep. "Okay," I told the room, "we can get to the next case."

I did it two more times that day: a bag of fentanyl was delivered and I switched it out with normal saline while pocketing the real thing. No one noticed or would even think to notice—anesthesiologists are constantly drawing up, hanging and pushing medications with no one to question it. The other two patients also woke up in pain but after a little dilaudid, they were fine.

Overall, diverting opiates was way too easy.

I KNOCKED on Van's backdoor window and waited five minutes before knocking again. He finally appeared and opened the door.

"I told you, if I don't come, you leave and come back another time."

"Why?" I said, looking over his shoulder.

"I'm not always available even when I'm home." He looked over his shoulder, back into his home.

I fidgeted with my feet, not knowing what he wanted me to do. I was in uncharted territory and had no idea how violent the guy was—I really didn't want to piss him off.

"What do you have for me?" he finally asked.

I opened up my backpack and took out the half liter bag of fentanyl, now unmarked.

His eyes almost popped out of his sockets like a cartoon character. "Is this what I think it is?"

I nodded.

He took the bag in his hands and cradled it in the crook of his elbow like it was a baby. "Very good." I took out the other two bags and I thought he was going to faint. "This is good. *Very* good." He looked incredibly relieved.

"How much do I get for each?"

His face soured. "I'll take care of it."

"Okay," I said, not knowing what he meant.

He took a step backward into his house and placed a hand on the door. "Come by tomorrow, same time." He shut the door.

"Okay," I said to no one, feeling both lonely and stupid.

I KEPT a low profile the next day at work and did some simple orthopedic cases—no diverting. I walked by the pharmacy window, trying to sense suspicious eyes on me—but it was a day just like any other. Lazlo kept clear of me and not a soul tried talking to me.

After leaving work, I got caught in the daily ritual of a twenty-minute traffic jam as everyone evacuated work at the exact same time. While waiting under a bridge, I glanced through the concrete column and saw scores of tents scattered throughout the underpasses of the freeway. Gnarled-hair vagrants milled around the encampment while tattooed teenagers moved from tent to tent, marauding and pushing people over. It was a Mad Max dystopia playing out alongside the snaking traffic of BMWs and Teslas. It was not a new scene to me, of course, but that day I wondered why all those people in that concrete jungle were there. Certainly they all had a story: bad home, bad boyfriend, bad school—bad dad. I pondered for a moment—or rationalized for a moment—were drugs the origin of their stories or merely the lubricant—the scapegoat? Surely drugs had become the currency of that tent town, but were they the cause of their woes?

I doubted it.

I doubted it even more when Van gave me forty two thousand dollars later that night.

"Did they get the money?" I asked Zella after she came home from work.

"Yes. It was just in time—said they were already trying to transfer her out today to another facility."

I'd given ten grand for Zella's mom's nursing facility. It hurt but I knew it would smooth things over—make her happy and things a little more liveable at home.

"Thank you for putting in more hours," she said, a new easiness to her voice.

"It has to be done."

"Feels good," she said.

"I know. Feels like we're on the upswing—that we can get out of this."

She took my hand and wrapped it around her shoulder. "I told you."

We went to the park the next day, the girls paddling along in one of those giant plastic sports cars. There was something about the breeze or glowing sunset that started to set into my bones—I actually felt good. Sudden and nearly uncontrollable urges of violence against Lazlo were evaporating. Zella didn't let go of my hand and Regina actually called me daddy as she stuck her head out of the tiny sunroof of her mock corvette. It was also one of those sweet moments in life where you forget about how much you hate lawyers.

There was a whisper, though, and it was Farrah. I imagined her watching me, knowing what I was doing—screaming at me from behind some ethereal one-way mirror—that I was the biggest fucking idiot of her entire life—and afterlife. That she'd wasted all of her efforts on a total, drug-diverting-screw-up as myself. I rebutted with the fact that she'd been doing it her entire career, to which she retorted that I was the reason that she killed herself.

Touché.

After packing up for the day, I took baby Kris in my arms, my eyes sweeping the area for anything we'd left behind.

And then I saw someone.

A man sitting opposite the monkey bars, seated at a bench. He either watched me or something beyond me—too dark and distant to discern his focus. I feigned as if I didn't notice him and looked back—he hadn't moved.

"Someone you know?" Zella asked.

"No, I—"

And then he stood, walking toward us. My heart beat faster and I didn't know why. I put Kris down, clenching my fists and setting my jaw. His feet crunched in the gravel of the playground as he honed directly in on us. I took mental notes: khaki pants, brown leather belt, sky-blue polo shirt—looked like every man at a mall trying to sell you a new cell phone plan. His face—

"Hey!" he shouted.

I pointed at myself like an idiot until a little girl went running past my legs.

"There you are!" he said, scooping the girl into his arms. "You're getting good at hiding," he told her, giving her nose a pinch. He looked at me, gave a smile and walked off.

And that's when I knew.

Paranoia was going to be my best friend.

CHAPTER FOURTEEN

"What—uh—what am I looking at here?" I asked the woman opposite the glass display case.

She swept a heavily tattooed arm across the display. "These are mostly Springfields and SR9s. I got some Browning High Powers at the back of the store you can look at."

"No—I mean—are these ones that I...would want?"

The woman cocked one eye at me. "Depends on why you want one."

"Like I said, personal protection."

"Then yes, a handgun—one of these here—would do fine." She held a smirk on her face letting me know she thought my white-bread attempts to buy a gun were adorable.

"So which should I get?"

"This one here," she said, tapping at the glass. "Glock 26. Easy to conceal, easy to use." She took it out of the case and laid it on a strip of red velvet fabric streaked with gun oil. It was small and blocky as if the thing was constructed of Lego bricks—it may as well have been—I certainly wouldn't have recognized the difference. I looked at her expectantly.

"Go ahead."

I picked it up, squeezing it in my fist.

None of it felt right. Me standing there—this Metallica-roadie gazing at me like she was a proud mother—Zella working, the girls at home with a nanny. And me: holding a gun, trying to figure out just who in the hell I was.

The gun-lady then brought out a shoulder holster and had me try it on, helping lift it over my arm. After putting the gun in the holster, she had me put my jacket on over it and move to the full body mirror.

"See?" she said, jabbing at my rib. "No one will notice a thing. But you will. You'll know you can handle anything that comes at you."

I paid in cash and, as I walked out of the store, realized I had no idea if she had done a criminal background check or anything on me. The whole affair had taken no more than twenty minutes. Apparently, when you're a white guy, getting a firearm is as easy as purchasing an umbrella.

I KEPT LOOKING in the rearview mirror as I drove to the shooting range. I couldn't stop thinking about Van's little party a few weeks prior. It was full of dubious looking characters. I was certain if any of them caught wind that Van's bestie next door neighbor was now supplying him boatloads of narcotics, I'd have a huge bull's eye painted on my back. I googled "how to know if you're being followed." I found some hot tips targeted at women trying to hide from stalkers but not a lot else for a novice drug dealer like myself.

After I fired off a few rounds at a flimsy sheet of paper in the shape of a would-be assailant, I looked at the gun in my hands. Even after firing, it still seemed so small—so insignificant. It was a bit of metal—some springs and cylinders—formed into a crucible of gunpowder and projectiles. It was a tool designed to bluntly take care of problems. It asked no permission and gave no apologies. After I fired a few more rounds I put it away. There was no high after shooting it—no sense of power like I'd heard about. It only made me feel thirty years older—gray hair, driving around in a Corvette with a twenty-year old blonde in the passenger side.

I WAS on trauma duty later that night—starting a string of night shifts. I was two steps into the shift and the Code Trauma alarm went off. After rushing down to the ER, I saw not one but two crowds of healthcare providers, huddled around two patients lying opposite one another in the resuscitation bay. It was near impossible to know what was going on—too many nurses yelling, too many interns looking helpless and too many doctors barking out orders that no one could hear. So, I elbowed my way to one bed and saw a man oozing with blood. Someone scattered a round of bullets into his belly. He had a pulse, a breathing tube and was getting five units of blood poured into his veins. After they sheared his clothes from his body, I saw that Old English font lettered across his chest and flanks. If that weren't sign enough of the thug-life, a few tear drop tattoos cusped the sides of his eyelids.

I made my way to the other bed and saw someone hopping up and down like they were on a pogo stick. A boy, no more than fourteen years, was bouncing up and down in the gurney with each chest compression. With every pump, blood spouted from his mouth, covering everyone. After getting to the top of the bed, I found an oozy mess clinging to his hair. Probing with my finger, I felt shattered skull and the soft sponge of brain tissue.

"Brain matter, here!" I yelled.

"Call it," The ER doc yelled, waving her hands like she was an umpire who'd just called a strikeout.

The compressions stopped and the boy collapsed back into bed—arms splayed, the spouting of blood turning to a gentle weeping. His eyes—like those glass orbs they put in stuffed animal eye sockets. We were all silent for a long moment, some likely pondering and lamenting the flame of life that had just been blown. And then I remembered the first guy still trying to die right next door.

The trauma surgeon yelled out, "Ex lap!" which mobilized the nurses. They got the patient packed up to go to the operating room. It meant the guy was bleeding out his guts, or liver or spleen—or wherever—and the surgeons were going to take a look under the hood.

A whispering commotion bubbled up around me: "...said he was the shooter...the kid was the target...gang related."

"What?" I asked one of the EMS agents standing next to me.

"That guy," he said, pointing at the gangster. "He shot the kid. Gang retaliation. The kid's brothers were right around the corner and shot him back."

"You sure?"

"We didn't exactly hang around to ask questions, but that's what it looked like, yeah."

"Let's go!" the surgeon yelled.

I stepped to the head of the gurney and wheeled the patient away, down to the ORs. Once there, I put in a large central line into his neck and continued pumping him full of blood and plasma as the belly continued to dump blood. The surgeons unzipped his belly with a scalpel and went elbow deep, rummaging around viscera and bowel. The patient's blood pressure started to tank—even after I started an infusion of epinephrine, norepinephrine and vasopressin. His heart rate was dropping.

"Guys," I told them, "we're losing him."

The nurse said something under her breath. I couldn't tell but it was something like *good riddance*.

"Suction!" the surgeon yelled followed by, "Gimme the clamp!"

And then there it was.

The blood pressure bumped up. He'd found the bleeder. After another hour, the removal of a spleen and kidney, the patient had finally stabilized. As the surgeons sewed up the man's belly, the black sutures criss crossed through his pallid skin.

We had just saved a child murderer.

Nothing new.

SEEMED like the right time to go on vacation.

Zella protested at first—said we couldn't afford it. But she was easy to break. I could tell working nights was getting to her—just being back to work after a few years hiatus was tough enough. Seeing the girls get excited to get on an airplane was reason enough for me.

"I'll be gone for a bit," I told Van after making a delivery on his back porch.

With a furtive glance around, he asked why.

"Vacation."

"That's it? Just a vacation?"

I nodded.

"Where are you going?"

"Why does that matter?"

He clicked his tongue after a moment of silence and came back with my payment. I flipped through the bills and gave him another nod.

So after sorting things out with my work, wife and drug distributor, we set off for San Diego. It was in a sweet spot of affordability that went a long way in convincing Zella. The weather was annoyingly perfect but I decided to not resent it and try to feel good for once. The ocean was immaculate as we laid out our implements for a day at the beach. For the first time in a while, I really wanted a beer—not to escape from my terrible situation but to enhance how incredible it was to let go for a few days. I resisted, as usual, and settled for a virgin mojito.

As I sucked on the tiny straw of my ridiculous drink, I noticed a bunch of skidrow-looking people conversing at the picnic tables. I knew the look—same people that dwelled under the freeway overpass outside my hospital. I knew who they were and I knew what they were doing. One gentleman opened a backpack between his legs and handed a baggie to another gentleman across from him. They made another exchange with their hands and, although I couldn't see the amount, I noticed several bills being passed. For the first time in my life, I was actually interested in what people like them were doing. Without a look back, the dealer left the picnic table and walked off. I stood, watching him go.

Zella looked up from her book. "Where you going?"

"Bathroom. Be back soon."

After slipping into my flip flops and bringing a sun visor over my eyes, I followed the guy. He lead me through downtown, past surfing shops and taquerias until he found a group of homeless women sitting near some dumpsters in an alley. I pretended to play on my phone as he made an exchange and then moved on. He walked methodically and made his way through the streets with precision—he had a route. After twenty minutes of following, he turned down a street corner and I lost him.

After looking for a moment, I turned to head back to the beach—

And then a pile of bricks fell on my head.

After being out for what felt only a moment, I realized the clobbering was indeed not a pile of errant bricks, but the fist of an angry drug dealer.

"Why you following me?" he hissed, spittle clinging to his lips.

"I'm...not."

"Who are you?"

He allowed me to get to my feet as I probed my face—my cheek bone was swelling up. With the horrible feeling that I was soon to be a patient at the nearest trauma hospital, I asked him, "How much?"

He looked me up and down, a smile cracking on his face. "*You*?"

"How much for fentanyl?"

"You must be the worst undercover I've ever seen."

"No—it's not that. I have a friend. She's dying of cancer—can't get any pain medications, so I'm looking to help her out."

"You playing?"

"Look I'm sorry, never mind." I turned but then heard him speak up.

"Fifty for a patch."

"A patch? You only have patches?"

He nodded. "I don't have any now. Meet me at this corner same time tomorrow."

"I will. Thank you."

He snorted at me and walked off.

Zella gaped at me when I returned to the beach. "What happened to your face!"

"Oh—I—got hit."

She jerked her head back, nonplussed and held out her arms, awaiting some sort of sane explanation.

"It was an accident. Some lady was opening an awning over a shop and—bam!—right in the face."

I tossed and turned that night in the hotel. After some savvy googling, I discovered that most dealers either sold shitty, impure fentanyl made in homebrewed labs or fentanyl patches stolen from the healthcare industry. The pure, pharmaceutical grade stuff I was delivering to Van on a silver platter rarely ever made it to the streets. A fentanyl patch—the kind a patient slaps on their skin for extended-release absorption—also had much less of the drug than the liquid form. After crunching some numbers I came to a shockingly unsurprising conclusion:

Van was screwing me over.

Royally.

On our last day of vacation, we got lunch on a patio overlooking the beaches. I was still sulking over how much I was risking to make Van a millionaire.

"Not yet," Regina said. She dug her index fingers into the corners of my mouth.

"Ow!"

"Vacation isn't over. No Doomy Gloomy Daddy yet."

"Oh—yeah." I gave her a quick smile which she didn't believe for a moment. She stuck her tongue out and then walked off to the beach.

I heard a voice to my left. "Kids."

I looked over at a man: straw-woven hat, Tommy Bahama shirt. Sandals—with white tube-socks. "Yeah," I said, not relishing the prospect of shooting the shit with a tourist.

"I got three at home," he said, reaching for his phone to show me unsolicited pictures.

"Nice," I said, giving a brief glance.

"They are a handful. Something I can see you're well acquainted with." Somehow, he took my non-committal grunts as a sign to pull up a chair. "You on vacation, too?"

"Yes."

"No business?"

"Nope."

"I'm visiting from a little town outside Chicago. You?"

"Seattle."

"Ha! Getting outta the rain are we?"

"Something like that." No matter how much I ignored eye contact, the man could not take a hint.

"So when you packing things up?"

"Leaving today actually." I stood and looked at my wrist, forgetting that I didn't wear a watch. "Whoo, looks like we better get going. Have a good one," I told him, sliding my hands into my pockets.

"You, too," he said, "you, too."

DIVERTING opiates had become just a normal part of my work

day. I would've been much more worried about it had I not known that Farrah had done it her entire career without once getting caught. I clocked in, did some cases, faked the medical record that I was giving fentanyl to a patient and just put it in my pocket. It was that easy. Thinking back to when I did it for Farrah—heart pounding, looking over my shoulder at the pharmacy bean counters—I'd become a reasonably cool cucumber about the whole operation.

I was too afraid to carry the gun around. Not in fear of the gun, but fear that Zella would give me a hug and suddenly notice that her husband was packing heat. The gun spent most of the time in a rusty, overturned wheelbarrow in the garage. I put it on under a jacket every time I had one of my dates with Van.

"Nothing more?" Van asked when I delivered him about two dozen vials of fentanyl.

It's not as if I enjoyed our arrangement. Despite my actions, I didn't exactly relish jeopardizing my career, family and risking jail time every single day I walked into work. But when I got an almost non-existent paycheck every two weeks, it was a nice reminder of why I was doing it. I'd also developed a convenient sense of justice every time I diverted: it was Lazlo's fault, hence the hospital's fault, that I was in dire financial straits.

With a bite in my voice, I told Van, "That's all I could get this week."

He considered the vials in his hands like they were spare change he was about to toss. "You can't get the half liter bags?" I could tell he was nervous about something.

"It's a delicate balance. It's not an a-la-carte thing. I take what I can depending on what I'm doing that day. If I push it too much, people will get suspicious."

"I could really make it worth your time if you can increase the volume."

"Does that mean you'll stop undercutting me?" I couldn't help it. I didn't want to push the man who held an incredible amount of leverage over me—but he was screwing me over.

He failed to hide his surprise. "What do you mean?"

"You know what I mean."

We shared an uncomfortable silence. A dangerous silence.

"Tell me what you want," he finally said.

"Fifty percent more."

"I'll see if I can get you twenty."

"You'll *see*? What do you need to do, go file the request with your district manager?"

"Bring me three half liter bags like last time."

"You'll get it in a week."

I DIDN'T EVEN HAVE to request doing spine cases—I was assigned the next day. I had four major spine operations and so I ordered four, half liter bags of fentanyl, one for each case. As I switched the labels in the operating room, I stared into the clear liquid—a certain awe spilling over me. At one time in my life, I would've been diverting to shoot the stuff up my veins—a thought that had become ludicrous.

The day ended late, but I had four golden geese hidden in my gym duffle bag as I walked out of the hospital. They would get me a lot of money—maybe enough to stop the ridiculous enterprise altogether. Yet, as I opened my car door, my hopes for earning upwards of a hundred grand were smashed as I noticed two men parked opposite me.

They were looking right at me.

They had been...waiting for me.

I stood paralyzed as the car doors opened simultaneously and two tall men in black suits emerged. Instinctively, I felt my chest wondering if by some miracle I strapped my gun on that day.

It wasn't there.

My mouth went dry as they approached, their hands going into their jacket pockets. As I was about to duck and squeal—realizing that I was a fraud in every aspect of my life including my new vocation of becoming a would-be, candy ass, drug kingpin—one of them spoke.

"Dr. Rosen?" the man on the left said.

"Yes?"

I flinched as he produced something from his pocket that was not a gun. It was a name badge. Three particular letters got my attention:

D, E and A.

"Mind if we ask you some questions?"

CHAPTER FIFTEEN

"How long have you been working as an anesthesiologist?"

I watched the two men opposite the shiny, metallic table that I thought was only reserved for Hollywood studios whenever someone was interrogated. The moment didn't seem real. Yes, I'd been "selling drugs", but what I was doing seemed so disconnected from my image of criminal activity. I simply took some liquid home from work and delivered it to my neighbor who happened to highly value that liquid and paid me accordingly. That was it. Did I really deserve to be sitting across from two middle aged-men in black suits who were so obviously trying to goodcop/badcop me?

"My partner asked you a question," the Badcop said. He had the permanent grimace of someone trying to hold in a fart.

"About fifteen years," I told them, my fingers interlaced, thumbs adjoining. I didn't know how to behave. I hadn't quite figured out which angle I should take: the indignant arrogant prick or the doe-eyed innocent family man. I was pretty sure neither would be convincing. The truth was I had no idea what I was doing and I was absolutely terrified. The foolishness of my decisions were creeping in: did I really think I could just sell opiates to my neighbor without a soul noticing? I wasn't some mastermind, I wasn't a drug lord—and I certainly wasn't Walter White.

"And you've been at your current employment for that same period of time?" the Goodcop asked.

"Yes." The room was so silent it was impossible not to hear me swallowing. I was a fraud, sitting across from them. I knew it. I had always been a fake—should never have been accepted to med school, never gotten into residency. I never should have fooled an incredible woman to marry and have children with me thinking she was building a life with a real person. At times, I'd even fooled myself—believed that I did actually know what I was doing. But at that moment, looking at the two vipers in suits across from me—it reminded me of the reality of who I was.

"We appreciate you coming in with us, Dr. Rosen," the Goodcop continued, "I know it's a little late and you'd like to get home. You got kids?" He smiled like a car salesman.

"Two."

"Ha, me too," he said, pulling out his phone and flipping through pics of his two dumb kids.

"Why am I here?"

Badcop said, "Because we have some questions to ask you and the current question has to do with the number of children you have. Is that a problem?"

"No. It's not a problem." I took a deep breath and tried not to let an ounce of my body language indicate that there were 2 liters of fentanyl sitting in my gym bag, under my chair. If they decided to search me at any moment that would be the end of my universe forever, amen.

Goodcop started. "We've been having issues, lately, Dr. Rosen, in the community with prescription narcotics."

"Right."

"You're aware?"

"Of course I'm aware. I'm a doctor with schedule II narcotic prescribing powers. It's my job to know."

"Oh yes, of course," he carried on as if we were neighbors talking over the fence while Badcop frowned at me. "Me and my partner here are tasked specifically with red-flagging and targeting prescription fraud committed by physicians. Did you know such a surveillance existed?"

"Of course."

"That's good, Dr. Rosen, because I'd like to hear from you why you believe we have brought you here today."

"What do you mean?"

"Clearly you've drawn our attention. I'd like to get your opinion. Why do you think we're sitting right here asking you questions this evening?"

Odd. They either knew everything or nothing. I wondered if Van was in another interrogation room, spilling his guts about his new supplier. I decided that they were going to have to squeeze every drop of information from me. "I have no idea," I told them.

"None?"

"No. I'm assuming I've been red-flagged for some reason. Why don't you tell me why that is?" I wondered if they could tell how sweaty my armpits were.

"We don't have to tell you shit," Badcop barked.

"Excuse me, gentlemen, but I don't see handcuffs on my

wrists so I don't think I'm under arrest. I think if you'd like to go around in circles with me then I'd best be getting home to my kids."

"That bruise on your cheek. Where'd you get it?"

"Vacation. San Diego."

"Why'd you go to San Diego?"

"I just told you. Vacation."

"Farrah Abdi," Badcop said.

I froze and they saw that I froze. What could the DEA possibly want with Farrah? Did they know about her diversion? "What about her?"

"Who is she to you?"

"My dead best friend. Thanks for asking."

They shared a furtive glance and the Goodcop said, "She died with a lot of opiates in her bloodstream."

"I know. She had cancer."

"Did you know she had an oncologist who was prescribing her pain medications?"

"Yes."

"Then why did you write a prescription for her, Dr. Rosen?" They threw a photocopy of a prescription with my stupid signature at the bottom.

Everything in my body unclenched. It was about Farrah—about the opiate prescription I'd written for her during her pain crisis. The DEA doesn't like it when physicians prescribe opiates to friends—makes them antsy.

"Oh. Okay," I said, "that's what this is about. Look, I'm sorry, okay? She was writhing in pain—breast cancer eating at her bones. Her oncologist refused to prescribe her more meds so I did it myself. You'll see—if you look—that I've never once prescribed outpatient opiates before or after."

They glanced at one another again. It was starting to get annoying. Their silence was encouraging—like they were trying to improvise after my unexpected admission. But then Goodcop grimaced and Badcop nodded. Shit. There was something more.

Goodcop said, "Do you know how she died?"

"Why are we talking about this?"

Badcop leaned forward. "Answer the question, doctor."

"Overdose."

"Uh huh," Goodcop said, as if expecting more from me.

"She killed herself. Decided to end things early. Which is actually legal in this state when someone is terminal."

"Legal only if those drugs are prescribed by a physician. Do you know what was found in her arm?"

I froze.

SHIT.

I'd done many incredibly stupid things up until that point and one of the first had caught up to me. When I found her there—her body a withered, dessicated husk of flesh—I collapsed at her bedside. I raged at the world and fate or whatever else and forgot—forgot to remove the syringe of fentanyl that was still sitting in her vein.

The exact fentanyl that I supplied her. Illegally.

"No," I said.

"Fentanyl."

I feigned surprise but felt their glares melt my innocent veil.

"We spoke with her hospice nurse—she was unaware of any IV pain medications in the home."

"Yeah?"

"You know, Dr. Rosen," Badcop said, "if the fentanyl were

supplied to her illegally and was the cause of her death, that would be homicide."

"So you think I gave it to her?"

Goodcop produced a small baggie containing several vials. I already knew what they were—the vials of fentanyl I'd brought to her. "We've matched the serial numbers on these vials and we found out where they came from. Care to guess?"

"My hospital?"

They both nodded, pleased they'd gotten to their punchline.

I had to get out of there.

Now.

"Excuse me, gentlemen, but I think I should be leaving. Probably shouldn't answer anything without a lawyer now. You know, since I'm being accused of murdering my best friend and all." I stood, hefting my gym bag full of fentanyl. "You do know that Farrah was also an employee at the same hospital, right?"

"Yes, well—"

"And that she could've just as easily taken all those vials for herself?"

"We're exploring all possibilities."

"I didn't give her anything, agents. She was my best friend. I wouldn't have done anything to harm her."

"So you wouldn't mind supplying your fingerprints to clear this all up?"

"No problem." I showed them two fingerprints—both from middle fingers—and walked out.

MY HEART POUNDED on the way home. It wasn't the same

adrenaline rush when I was cutting open someone's trachea or wading through pools of blood to get someone breathing again. This was one of those clammy panics—the feeling of stepping up the ladder to an enormous diving board. I was in way over my head and should've recognized it long before I was sitting across from two DEA agents. More unnerving was that they were just finding out about the stuff I'd done months ago—crimes I was too clueless to know that I'd actually committed. Could they follow the trail to what I was doing now? What if they were also investigating my suspiciously rich neighbor?

I marched over to Van's and knocked on the back sliding door. A few moments later, he appeared. "What've you got for me?"

"Here," I said, dumping the liters of fentanyl into his arms. "Take it."

He quickly absconded with the goods and came back with some fat stacks. "A deal's a deal, Dr. Rosen."

I flipped through the bills. "How much?"

"Eighty large."

"Great, thanks." I slipped off the porch but he called out.

"Any more coming soon?"

I looked around the dark yard, peering into the streets. "No. Not for a while."

"You getting soft, now? Right when you're about to really start raking it in?"

"It's my wife—she's asking questions. I need to lay low for a bit."

"Okay next time let's just make it a cool one hundred for you. Sound good?"

"Fine, fine," I said marching off through the grass, "I'll let you know."

"I DON'T WANT A 'FOR SALE' sign on the property," I told the real estate agent. Both her and Zella gave me confused looks.

"Why not?"

"No advertising either. I want you to discreetly find a buyer. We'll take the asking price—or even lower. We need to sell inside a week." I had already pushed it far enough with Zella that week, insisting that we move. I'd made a good case for the move—we were now more solvent, we should rent someplace else for cheap to stay afloat, maybe she could stop working…All of these arguments were actually true—they just weren't the whole truth.

"One week?" Zella said. "I think we can take a little more time than that."

The realtor nodded in agreement. "Mr. Rosen, I think we need to see the market potential with your home. The market is hot right now and I think you can get at least fifteen percent over the asking price."

"No. We need to get out—out of the neighborhood."

"Why the rush?"

I asked the realtor to excuse us a moment. She left the room perplexed. "We need to sell fast," I told Zella.

"But shouldn't we take our time? Get the best asking price?"

"No—I…" I had gotten fairly decent at lying but I didn't know how to cover the real reason I wanted to leave.

Zella asked, "Are you worried that some of the equity will get seized?"

"Yes. Exactly. If we wait too long, the court will figure out and take a percentage of the sale." I didn't actually know if that was true. For all the gouging the court had done to me, I would've been surprised if it weren't true.

"What about the kids?"

"What about them?"

"They were raised in this home. We brought them home from the hospital here."

"This makes the most financial sense. We'll get equity out of our current home and save money by paying cheaper rent somewhere. We're only now starting to climb out of the hole we're in. If we downsize just a little more, we could get back on our feet."

She started to nod.

"And besides, we can move a little closer to your mom."

Her eyes lit up.

I had yet again successfully manipulated my wife.

I HADN'T HEARD from the DEA for over a week. I still wasn't entirely sure why they brought me in. Did they suspect I was behind Farrah's death or was it deeper? Were they just trying to scare a doctor who got a little too loose with his prescription pad? Or had they noticed a surge in medical grade fentanyl on the streets and were grasping at any red flags they could find?

I didn't sleep—didn't eat. A sharp pain in my belly signaled impending gastric ulcers from all the stress acid building up. I got calls—a lot of calls. Lots of them just hung up on me from numbers I didn't recognize. Gross tried talking to me even though I had nothing to say. Despite already having one lawyer, another woman was constantly trying to get me on my phone, leaving voicemails about how her firm needed to get in touch.

I couldn't handle any of it.

I found myself standing at the living room window. Watching. Waiting. For what? A SWAT team or a rival drug gang—either was possible at that point in my life. When I wasn't at the window, I found excuses to do yard work—yelling at Regina to get inside the house when she wanted to play around me. There was something deeply unsettling about watching your daughter play hopscotch on the sidewalk while you carried a firearm inside your jacket.

True to her word, our realtor didn't put up a sign—didn't do any advertising whatsoever. We found a buyer almost instantly who offered a little above our asking price. After signing the papers, we arranged for a moving company who guaranteed they could move the entire home in one day before noon.

I stood as a sentinel as seven movers brought out furniture and boxes—Zella watching me watching them. She carried a confused silence with her that week. I could tell gears were turning in her mind—certain that she should be suspicious of me but not knowing exactly why. As the morning dragged on, I kept one eye on Van's place—there was no movement, no lights. The streets, too, were quite: no nosey DEA agents wondering just what in the hell I was doing. When I came out from a bathroom break, I stopped short at the porch—

Van was talking to Zella.

"Hey!" I offered, wrapping my arm around Zella's shoulder. "What're you doing here?" I asked Van.

"You guys are moving?"

"Uuh…" I stalled, trying to think of any other believable reason why people were removing every item from our house. "Estate sale, actually."

Zella laughed. "You haven't told our neighbors we're moving?"

Van scrunched his nose. "Where to?"

"Burien," Zella answered before I could cut her off.

"Oh, good," Van said, "so not too far away. That's great for you guys."

"Van, do you mind if I come over right now and get my gym bag that I left at your house?"

He paused and then said, "Sure."

Once we were in the confines of his foyer, his face flattened. "What are you doing?"

"Moving."

"And why didn't you tell me?"

"I'm done."

"You're *what*?"

"This," I said, gesturing between me and him, "this is finished."

He took a deep breath. "You should've told me you were moving."

"Did you hear what I said? Our business arrangement has come to a conclusion." I turned, grabbed the door handle.

"Jude. This is a really bad idea." He had never called me by my first name before. There was something terrifying about it.

"No. Starting all of this with you was a bad idea."

"What spooked you?"

I wasn't about to tell him about the DEA. If the guy knew the DEA had brought me in just a few days prior, I'm pretty sure he'd have me murdered instantly. "Nothing. I'm just done with this. I appreciate you getting me out of a hole, but I don't need to do this anymore."

"No." He sighed. "You don't understand. You can't just stop like this. Just trust me, it is for your own good that you stay here. You don't have to keep supplying me forever—we can taper things down. Disrupting the market like this has consequences."

It was a threat, no doubt. But there was something more in his words than just intimidation. I opened the door and stepped out. "I'm never going to see you again. If you follow us, I'll...do bad things to you." A tangible threat, it was not.

I slammed the door.

CHAPTER SIXTEEN

We'd rented an outdated disaster made in the early nineties. The kitchen had peeled, lime-green linoleum flooring and the carpet was eternally redolent of cigarette smoke. The two bedrooms afforded us little silence—a fact of which Regina made abundantly clear as she "practiced" on her recorder.

The house was surrounded by trees. Tall trees. Thick trees. Trees that could make you feel like you're not continuously surveilled by drug enforcement or drug enforcers. Once we got everything moved in, I was already feeling better. Threatening Van felt wrong, but I only meant it as the final cherry on top of our break-up. I wanted him to know I was serious about ending my stint in the drug trade. I'd already risked too much up until that point. It was the perfect time to get out before I'd gone too deep.

Apparently, no one had told the hospital that the DEA had taken an interest in me, as my name kept popping up on the OR board for work. I showed up, did my cases, got my wages garnished, and went home. Besides getting away from the drug world I had slipped into, moving was the right thing for us. Zella continued working, and with less of a mortgage, we actually started getting our savings going again. Her mom was close by in a skilled nursing facility—to which we made payments on time. Regina was royally pissed about starting at a new school—but she had become impossible to please in any way lately so I took it as a net even. I took Zella out often—found a great park on the Sound for the kids to play. Even our dog seemed to be having the time of his life in the woods.

Everything was fine.

It all worked out.

The end.

I'D FOUND Regina's bike in the garage, overturned, with the chain dangling off the gear. Normally, she would've come running to me to fix it but since the move to a new house, she kept a distance. Even worse, she'd just sit through story time like an obligatory staff meeting she had to attend: silent, arms crossed—waiting for me to finish the story. The growing gap between us was more than alarming. Trying to have some sort of semblance as a father was one of the few things that kept my head above the insanity.

As I crouched beside her tiny bike, W-40 in hand, a shadow darkened the open garage. When I looked up, I saw only the silhouette of a man—the morning sun outlining his figure. He kept one arm to his side as if he were carrying something—or concealing something in his shirt.

"Hello?" I said, bringing a hand to my brow.

"Good morning," he said.

I stood, accidentally dropping the W-40 to the ground, the

ricochet sounding like gunfire against the concrete. "Can I help you?"

As he stepped into the garage, blood pumped into my head. I tensed, steeling myself for some sort of showdown against the harbinger of my bad deeds.

As the glare of the sun vanished, his face became clear. "You're new in the neighborhood?" he asked. I relaxed as I discovered the most benign man I'd ever seen: short brown hair, blue polo shirt tucked into pleated dockers. I felt even more ridiculous when the thing I thought he'd been concealing was, in fact, a baby.

"Yeah," I told him, "we moved in a few weeks ago. You're in the neighborhood, too?"

He smiled and said, "No," bouncing the baby up and down.

"Oh. Well who is this little guy?" I asked, pointing at the baby. It felt good to have a normal conversation with someone for once in which I wasn't trying to manipulate the situation. It made me realize I'd probably become a horrible person.

"I think his name is Adam," he said, rubbing the child's foot.

"You *think*?"

He nodded. "I believe so, yes. I'm just watching him."

"Oh…"

"Where did you move from?"

"From in town. Not far."

"Is that your little girl's?" he asked, motioning to the bike.

I nodded. "Yeah, so if you'll excuse me, I better fix it or she'll kill me."

He laughed and said, "Well I wouldn't want that to happen."

"Nice to meet you," I said, looking at his face, realizing there was something familiar about him. It was like hearing a familiar song or watching a scene from a movie but you're not quite sure how you know it. Quickly, an unease sprouted from my belly.

"I better get going," he said, "need to get little Adam here back. His daddy is a client of mine."

"Hmph." I squatted back next to the bike, wishing the man would vanish.

"You're also a client of mine, Dr. Rosen."

I stood, holding my breath. "*What*?"

He smiled, exposing a wide set of perfect, white teeth. "You work for me."

"What are you talking about?"

"You work for me," he repeated, his face drained of any humor.

A long silence.

"I have no idea what you're saying. I think you should get off my property now."

"Don't worry," he said, "everything will be fine."

"Who the hell are you?"

He turned, walking back down the driveway. "I'm nobody to you. You're going to want to keep me a nobody."

He walked off, happily bouncing the baby in his arms.

I WAS bloodshot tired the next day at work—no sleep happened for me. I stayed awake in the living room, looking out the blinds and watching for the darkening presence of someone walking by the streetlights. I couldn't get the guy's face out of my mind yet—I also couldn't remember what he looked like in a line-up. Despite having the most forgettable, suburban appearance of anyone I'd ever seen—I knew I had seen him before. All throughout my OR cases that day, I kept trying to picture his face but could only remember his teeth beneath a tiny snarl—a certain impatience and danger well concealed but readily unleashed.

My first instinct was to move. Again.

But not only would Zella not go for that, I was pretty sure whoever this guy was, he could just as easily follow me again. He'd known about me—knew what I was doing with Van. Despite my attempts to conceal our move, I wasn't exactly covert. My house could've been surveilled by anyone. As soon as the movers came, the trucks could easily have been followed. It was naive of me to think I could just leave behind a life of a being a drug supplier by making a small move across town. I had been beyond dumb, but I sure as hell wasn't going to start supplying some guy who showed up on my doorstep.

I had to do something.

My first thought was going to the DEA. It would be so easy. Just show up, confess the whole thing—tell them some new distributor was onto me—set up a sting to get the guy and it would all be over.

Except I'd be in jail for a very long time. My girls would grow up without a father and Zella would be alone to take care of them along with her dying mother. With no money. I wasn't about to let that happen.

My second thought was less savory. It involved keeping a gun on me and waiting for the guy to come sniffing around again. Did he really think he could just show up to my house and start demanding things without a little push back?

As these things rolled around in my mind—the DEA, jail time, my fatherless children—I walked across the parking garage at the hospital and stopped.

There he was.

Leaning against my car.

"Dr. Rosen," he said, that smile creeping up his face, "so nice to see you again." He was wearing a navy blue jumpsuit fitted with a reflective safety vest. The ensemble was complete with a streak of grease across his brow. He looked like someone who'd worked in maintenance his entire existence. Earlier with the polo shirt and khakis I'd thought him Caucasian with some eastern European blood but now—in the uniform of the working class—he looked Filipino. He was like an ethnic chameleon.

My hand went to the gun hidden inside my jacket.

He shook his head, pointing at my hand. "So...you think I work alone?"

I set my jaw, anger boiling inside.

"That piece won't keep anyone safe," he said, moving away from my car. "Here, let me get this for you." He opened my car door, despite it being previously locked.

I didn't move.

"I know you've been busy with the move. I'll give you a few more days before we start doing business." He receded away, into the darkness of the parking garage. "Have a safe drive home, Dr. Rosen."

"I GOTTA COVER a colleague for a few more hours," I told Zella over the phone, "won't be home until later."

"Is everything okay?"

I told her everything was fine, that there was nothing to worry about.

And then she asked me a question—a question that had obviously been churning in her mind. "Why are you...different?"

Feigning surprise was the only defense I could think of. "What do you mean?"

"Feels like you're not being honest with me."

"Being honest about what?" Honing in on what information an accuser has against you is the hallmark of a liar. Zella knew that.

"I think I've been putting up with a lot, lately."

I wasn't at all prepared to have the conversation she was attempting. "I know—with the move and going back to work. I've been asking a lot from you."

"No. Not that. You've been lying to me. Are you...using again?"

"Never," I told her. "That's ridiculous."

"You've been spending more time at work—working later…"

"It's only been for us, to help our family. I've been doing it all for you and the girls. I am not using, I swear it."

There was silence and then, "Okay."

I told myself that I'd make it up to her—make everything better again.

I got off the phone with her and drove to our old neighborhood. Our old house glowed with warm light in the twilight of dusk. I thought about how we'd brought home two beautiful baby girls through the front door—watched them grow. It had mostly been a home of warmth and happiness—something I wasn't entirely sure I could ever get back.

As I neared Van's house, I stopped short when I saw a "For Sale" sign sticking up through a mound of freshly turned dirt. The lights were off. Nothing stirred within.

"He moved?" I said to the crickets.

I walked up the porch with my hand on my gun, looking

over my shoulder. I knocked on the front door and knocked again. After no answer, I knocked for thirty seconds straight.

Nothing.

The moment I get out of the game and move, a new stranger appears—demanding I supply him with not-so-subtle hints of what would happen if I didn't. And now, the only person who was directly linked suddenly decided to sell his home and disappear? It was all delightfully ominous.

"No," I said to the night as I walked to the backyard, "nuh uh." I approached the sliding window door—the same door where we'd had our exchanges. I saw my reflection in the moonlight. I looked weird and scared and alone. Shrugging that off, I tried the handle which was of course locked.

So I threw a rock through the door and walked in.

"Van!" I yelled, "Where the fuck are you!"

As the security alarm blared, I walked from room to room—gun out—discovering a fully furnished home—he hadn't moved yet.

"Who did you send after me?" I yelled, finding more empty rooms.

The place was immaculately clean.

I made my way upstairs, into the master bedroom, and found an armchair turned away from the doorway—turned for someone to watch the street.

And there he was.

That white smile turned—his dark eyes locking to mine. "Dr. Rosen."

I almost shot him out of sheer surprise.

"It's best you put the gun down," he said, "you won't find your old distributor here anymore. Seems he ran off on me. I do wonder how long he'll survive in the jungle." He stood, revealing dark, form fitting clothing like he was ready to rob a bank at midnight.

I took a step back.

How?

"I said, put the gun *down*."

I obeyed.

"Keep it, if you like, but it will do you no good. Your family's wellbeing is directly tied to my own. I thought I'd made that clear."

I couldn't respond. My mouth was bone dry. I was standing in front of a real-life-movie-villain—I had never been more petrified in my entire life.

He walked to the doorway, picked at the molding and said, "Come to Pike Place Market next Wednesday at 1 p.m. Do not appear empty handed. And I suggest you leave. Alarms bring police. Police make me...nervous."

And then he disappeared.

IT WAS all turning into some Greek tragedy.

I did at moments stop and ask myself: how could you have let this happen? How could you endanger your family like this? But did it matter why a drug lord now had a leash and collar wrapped around my neck? Would performing a root-cause analysis keep the gangsters from my girls?

I don't ask these questions anymore.

Not only because they're stupid questions but mostly because they don't matter.

The answer, of course, was that everything was my fault—but I knew that all along. I had no delusions about my motivations or about what I was doing. I felt justified because never in my life did I really believe I was someone who was...good. There were times—years even—where I felt like a normal, well balanced individual. I actually believed at one point that I deserved Zella—earned the life that was given to me. But now, with everything hanging on by a thread—Farrah gone, bankruptcy, the DEA and now dangerous people after me—things finally made sense.

This is who I was.

Jude the parasite.

It was almost liberating.

I got myself into it—only I could dig myself out.

CHAPTER SEVENTEEN

Each day I showed up for work, I was always surprised to see my name on the OR board. I was still a doctor—still a trusted individual to provide medical care to helpless people. Somehow, nothing of my real self had leaked into my professional career.

Yet.

Lazlo looked at me and nodded. He was right about me all along—suspicious of me even back when I was a resident, shooting up in the call room. He was the only one who knew to get rid of me—that I was a cancer within the system. If only Farrah wasn't naive enough to think I could change, I would've been caught—thrown out of residency. I never would've met Zella and destroyed her life. I'd probably be living in an alley somewhere—if I were even still alive.

I did a couple of plastic surgery cases that day.

Long and boring.

Plenty of time to think about the smoking crater that had become my life.

I held a few vials of fentanyl in my hands, turning them

side to side and watching the clear liquid swirl against the glass. So much of my life had revolved around the drug: giving pain relief to patients, self-medicating my emotions, providing release to my best friend, making tens of thousands of dollars —both as a physician and as a drug dealer. And now, my girls' lives depended on supplying it to a drug lord.

How did he know?

How could this man intercept my life three times in twenty four hours? He knew everything about me—knew where I'd go and what I'd do. He knew we had moved—knew I'd go to Van's after threatening me in the parking garage. How long was he following me—?

And then I remembered that face: small, sharp angles, both stoic and friendly.

I'd seen it before—months before. But where? Knowing he was associated with Van, I combed my memory of every interaction I had with the freakshow of party guests that graced his home. And then I remembered: there was a hipster staring at me from across the party, watching me—analyzing me.

And then the scrolls of my memory unfurled.

I'd seen him at the park while playing with the girls. He was dressed like a cell phone salesman, chasing his daughter around. He was the same man from San Diego—the tourist, showing me pictures of his kids on his phone, wondering why I was visiting. It was so obvious why he would follow me there —wondering if I had a new contact at the border. He'd been watching me the whole time—the boss behind Van's operation.

He was a chameleon—inserting himself into any social setting, hiding in plain sight.

Waiting.

Planning.

It seemed so obvious now. I was a cash cow to someone

like him. What better person to threaten and blackmail than a whitebread, suburban doctor desperate for some cash? Better yet, if I tried to turn on him, I'd go to jail for the rest of my life. He didn't show his face as I played by the rules, but once I tried to get out—he reveals himself.

And he wasn't going to let me go easily.

I SHOWED up at Pike Place Market.

Scores of tourists sifted through kiosks and rows of flower shops. They lined the fish market, shouting with glee as the men flung enormous fish over their heads. The air was full of fresh donuts and fried seafood. I'd brought the girls for Saturday morning breakfast and shopping a thousand times before. It was one of the most crowded and liveliest spots in the city—

And probably the worst place in the world to exchange drugs for money. Was the guy dumb or arrogant? After walking up and down the market, I found a spot next to the enormous golden piggy bank and waited for about an hour.

The Chameleon didn't come.

After waiting another thirty minutes, I left. I called Zella as I drove home. "Everything okay?"

"Yeah. Why?"

"No reason. Just checking in."

"Where are you?"

"I was at work. Driving home now."

"No, you weren't."

"I—"

"I called. They said you weren't on the schedule."

"I was doing paperwork in my office."

"You're sure?"

"Yes—hang on. I'm getting another call."

She hung up without another word.

"Hello?"

"Go back," a voice said.

"Who is this?"

"Go back." The line went dead.

I parked and returned to the market, more annoyed than scared. I waited once again and saw no one but families and couples on dates.

"Good afternoon, Dr. Rosen," someone said next to me. It was the Chameleon. Standing...right next to me. I hadn't noticed him because he was behind a baby stroller, a woman standing at his side.

"Oh. Hello," I said, not knowing how to proceed or what to do with my hands.

The baby in the stroller was different from the one he had when he visited my garage. The woman on his arm was silent, her eyes criss-crossing the crowds. Her mascara was a mess, streaking down her cheeks. She then looked at me, some sort of pleading in her face.

"Dr. Rosen this is Macey," the Chameleon said. "Say hello," he told her.

"Hello," she said and looked away.

"She and little Jason here were kind enough to join me for a little walk in the market today. Her husband is out doing some errands for me, so I said I'd take care of them while he was away—make sure they were safe while he did exactly what I told him to do. Macey and Jason don't have anything to worry about. They'll get home safely tonight as long as her husband doesn't try to do anything against my explicit instructions again."

The guy was insane.

I wasn't used to his level of crazy. Sure, I'd seen the consequence of psychopaths in the ER—people shot up in gang fights or stabbed half to death. But the Chameleon was next level stuff. Kidnapping someone's family and masquerading as the father in order to intimidate your next victim? I suddenly missed Van—my friendly drug dealer next door. Never would I had started this game had I'd known I'd unleash this kind of inhuman sociopath into my life.

"What took so long?" I asked.

"Had to watch you."

"You watched me sit here for an hour?"

He nodded. "And watch for a sting."

The guy was beyond careful.

"Here," I said, shoving a paper bag at him.

He glared at me, making his displeasure known that I was trying to run the meet and greet. Cradling the bag in his palm, he opened it and looked in. A flat smile spread across his face and he returned the bag to me. "No."

"No?"

"This is not good enough."

"Yes. It is."

"I see."

"What?"

"You believe you're still in charge. Perhaps I've been too subtle about what I will do to you if you don't obey."

"This is all I could get—"

"You will bring me ten liters of fentanyl at fifty micrograms per cubic centimeter. What you've brought is not even one percent of that amount."

"I can't get that much at a time."

"Either you can or you can't. There will be consequences either way."

"It's not possible."

He turned to the woman. "Macey, shall we be going?" She nodded and looked down at her child, rubbing his hand. The three started moving through the crowds.

"I can't do it!" I yelled.

He heard me.

But I had a feeling he didn't care.

"LAZLO, I'd like to do some spinal cases tomorrow." Amazing that I used to think Lazlo was my enemy. I had no idea what making an enemy really meant before becoming acquainted with the Chameleon.

"That's fine," he said, penciling it in on the schedule the next day.

"Do you mind putting me in spine rooms for the rest of the week?"

"Why?"

"I'm going to start a clinical trial."

"Oh, yes. I heard about that. Something about fentanyl infusions?" He raised an eyebrow at me and I had no idea if it was out of suspicion or actual intrigue. Had the DEA spoken to him?

"I think by using fentanyl infusions during spine cases it gets ahead of the post-surgical pain—cuts down on postoperative opiate requirements. I hope to start the study soon I just want to see how I can protocolize it."

"Sounds interesting."

It was a huge relief. Spine cases were the only legitimate way to get a few liters of fentanyl at a time without pharmacy getting suspicious.

The next day I showed up at the pharmacy window. "I'm

doing three spine cases today, I'll need a half liter of fentanyl for each case."

The pharmacist shook her head. "I'm afraid not."

"What? Why?"

"New policy. We're no longer distributing high quantities of fentanyl for clinical use."

"What are you talking about? That's ridiculous. I need fentanyl infusions for my patient's today."

She shrugged. "Above my paygrade. Some top down decision made last week."

I found Lazlo at the OR front desk. "You hear anything about not being able to get fentanyl infusions from pharmacy?"

"Actually yes—had a meeting yesterday. Apparently the DEA has issued a county-wide recommendation that all hospitals in the area limit the distribution of high volume opiates to physicians and nurses."

"*Shit.*"

"Problem?"

"I...can't do my study anymore."

"I suppose not. You'll have to find something else to do."

EACH DAY, I walked by pharmacy, peeking in—trying to figure out where they kept different medications. But I couldn't see anything from their little bank-teller window.

As I unlocked my lock box full of dilaudid and midazolam, I looked at the vials—usually thinking them to be so much at once—but now, it was only a drop in the bucket of what I needed. Within the electronic kiosk, there were twenty of the lock boxes available each morning for each anesthesiologist to remove and use for the day. Even if I managed to steal every one of them—it still wouldn't be enough for the Chameleon.

Plus, I would certainly be caught trying to steal that much at once.

Desperation crept within me like a cold, rising tide.

The next day I showed up at the pharmacy window again. "Good morning, I'm doing a craniotomy for a pituitary tumor. Do you guys have DDAVP back there?"

"Hmm," she said, tapping her lips. She started looking around. "Maybe...do you need it right now?"

"I'd like it available in case the patient goes into diabetes insipidus during the case. It's happened to me once before and I was glad to have it immediately available."

"I'll have to look around for a bit."

"That's okay." I waited at the window until a pharmacy tech came through the security door of the pharmacy. I grabbed the door handle. "I can help you look," I said as I came into the pharmacy work space.

She turned and looked at me with surprise. "That's not necessary."

"No, really, I know where you usually keep it." I pointed to a shelf in the back and followed behind her. Quickly, I glanced around the shelves and saw them sitting there like bars of gold: half liter bags of fentanyl, sitting on a top shelf.

"Here they are," she said, grabbing a vial of the medication that I really didn't need. "Why don't you come back around to the window and I'll scan this out to you?"

"Of course." As I turned to leave, I pulled out a strip of duct tape fitted with a thin piece of cardboard. After opening the door, I slapped the piece of tape over the strike plate in the door frame—covering the space where the door locks. I was deeply satisfied at the absent sound of the door locking into place as it closed.

"Thank you," I said, walking away.

I WAS ON NIGHT SHIFT.

Running between traumas in the ER and doing anesthesia for a hand amputation and emergent femur fracture in the ORs, I waited for down time. Once the ER was quiet and I had two residents in ORs doing my cases, I changed clothing in the locker room—knowing there were no security cameras there. In an old pair of jeans, red baseball cap and a denim jacket I'd bought at the Salvation Army the day before, I slipped down into the sterile hallways of the ORs and made my way to the unmanned pharmacy office. If I ran into any staff, they would've thought I was an idiot family member of a patient, and yelled at me to get out of the sterile, restricted area. But the halls were dark, quiet. With my jacket collar flipped up, and hat covering my head, I kept my face toward the ground, away from the hallway cameras that could later be audited.

I found the pharmacy door and pushed. It opened without resistance, my cardboard still covering the strike plate. The pharmacy was dark. I kept low, searching. I found a stack of half liter bags of normal saline and laid them on the ground. I then found the bags of fentanyl on a top shelf—there were eight of them. Four liters in total. I brought them down and started swapping labels. Carefully, I peeled the adhesive away with alcohol swabs from the fentanyl bags and then reapplied them to identical bags of saline with a new application of adhesive glue. After I finished I looked at the final product: they looked identical to the original. I put the dummy bags on the shelf and stepped back.

No one would notice the difference.

My hope was that they wouldn't even be used with the new hospital policy prohibiting distribution of large volume opiates. They would sit and collect dust. Even if they were used—say during an operation—it was possible no one would even find out they were fake if they were given to a fully anesthetized patient—someone unable to tell you if they're "feeling it". It was possible that the frauds would be discovered and then they would use spectroscopy on the fluid, discovering that it was nothing but saline. They would then look at the camera footage and see me—some random, criminal yokel who never looked up at the camera.

It was all incredibly risky. But that's what every move in my life had become: a colossal risk. It didn't matter in what direction I moved, it was a risk-benefit analysis. The risk being death or jail, the benefit being life with my family.

It was a plan that could possibly work—

Could work if a thousand assumptions aligned in a single celestial event.

He found me.

I never had to worry about that.

I wouldn't have been surprised if he put a GPS tracker on my car, clothing or straight into my cerebellum. I didn't even bother searching for a tracker—it would just piss him off if I found and destroyed it. I was at a gas station, filling up. He pulled up alongside me, rolled down his window and said, "The Troll. Tomorrow at 3pm."

I met him there the next day. A massive concrete troll statue made as if crawling out from the underside of a bridge overpass. It was another Seattle tourist hotspot. Apparently the Chameleon liked doing his business in the open. Easy access to hostages if things went wrong? I didn't want to find out.

I waited at the foot of the statue, the fentanyl stacked

within a Trader Joe's tote bag at my feet. It took another hour until he showed, dressed in jeans, an AC/DC t-shirt with a thin, leather jacket. Thankfully he was alone.

"Here," I said, handing him the bag.

"Smile, Dr. Rosen. We're friends who are just running into one another." It explained the outfit. He was trying to appear in my demographic.

I gave him the cheesiest smile of my life and said, "That's all I could get."

He opened the bag and looked at me. "More."

"No. There wasn't anymore. That's it."

"Please," he said, "explain in detail why you failed."

"I can't get what I used to for Van. What you're holding right there I had to steal outright—this is going beyond simple diverting. It's no longer available. If I keep trying to get it, I'm going to get caught and it's going to lead straight back to you. This is our last meeting—this is all you're going to get. I'll even waive the fee in good faith. Just take it."

"You'll...waive the fee?"

I nodded.

"You thought you were getting *paid*?"

"I—"

"I'm...disappointed, Dr. Rosen. It's my fault in assuming you understood our arrangement."

"What arrangement?"

He bared his white teeth and said, "You are a slave."

"*What?*"

"I am your master and you do as I say."

"You—"

"You think I...*need* you? That I *need* your supply—?"

"I'll go to the police."

He went silent—temples rippling as his jaw clenched.

My cheeks suddenly felt hot. "Take it. We can just go our separate ways."

He threw the bag of fentanyl at my feet and backed away.

"What're you doing?"

"The street value at your feet is half a million," he said.

"And?"

He continued staring at me.

"*And?*"

"I was showing you mercy by only making you a supplier. Now to demonstrate your worth, you're now the supplier, the distributor and street hustle. I expect payment in a week."

"Are you *crazy*? I can't move all *this!*"

"You're probably right," he said, flipping out his phone. "It is a shame," he said more to himself than anyone, "I thought he was smarter than the others."

"You'll just have to kill me," I told him.

He said that would also be fine and then left in an Uber.

CHAPTER EIGHTEEN

I showed up at work the next day.

There was no commotion—no whisperings about a robbery in the pharmacy. As I passed by the window, I looked in and saw my dummy bags of fentanyl sitting on the top shelf, undisturbed. It was then that I also realized my fingerprints were all over the bags. I wasn't exactly cut out for the thug life. Turns out it required far less intellect to be an anesthesiologist than to run a criminal enterprise. I was miserable proof of that.

I'd put the problem out of my head all day, vacillating between the dazzling life choices that were laid before me. Stuck in downtown traffic slog gave me ample time to remember the Chameleon—the way he shrugged at my suggestion that he just kill me. It was really no problem for him. I would either hit the streets myself and come up with half a million or just wrap my lips around the barrel of his gun. He seemed okay with either outcome.

Once it was my turn to wait at the next red light for the following ten minutes, I looked out the window—to the freeway underpasses. Columns of concrete and exposed rebar stood as sentinels over a homeless encampment that weaved throughout the city like a hidden valley in some fantasy novel. It was like the Shire only with schizophrenics and drug addicts.

I parked illegally and set out on foot.

Rows of tents hugged rusted chain-links, nestled among mounds of trash and broken furniture. There were many high-quality tents whose occupants were dressed with the cleanliness and fashion you'd find at the mall—one degree removed from middle class. I found many hollow-cheeked, nicotine stained faces peering out at me as if I were there to perform their exorcism. I felt an enormous bastard. Not only had I profited from their lifestyle but barely side-stepped becoming one of them. Walking among them, my villainy was complete—

Well, not quite.

"Hey," I said to a woman I'd found laying inside a filthy sleeping bag.

She opened her eyes and said something like, "Muh?"

"Can I ask you a question?"

She looked at me like I was an alien who'd just landed, wanting to sell her insurance.

"Can you tell me where you get your…supply?"

I believe she literally chomped her teeth at me and rolled over. After I asked another man, all eyes were on me. It wasn't a great place to suddenly become popular. I knew how incredibly stupid it was but I was desperate. I figured I already had a very dangerous man threaten to kill me, what's the harm in a few more?

"Dr. Rosen," someone said behind me.

I flinched and saw a man sitting in a plastic lawn chair. Bits of twigs and leaves clung to his short beard. Street grim had worked its way into his clothes—but I still recognized him.

It was Van.

I wanted to be angry at him, but I was just relieved to see my neighbor alive. "What are you doing here?" I asked him, "And...why did you leave?"

He gave a morose smile, exposing much more skull at his temples. He'd lost weight. "He's after you."

I nodded.

"Wish you'd told me you wanted out."

"Why?"

"We could've planned it out together. Getting away."

"Getting away?"

"From him."

"Why can't you just walk away?"

"He's pure...business."

"I can't reason with him—ever?"

He shook his head. "We're all just resources. Once you're no longer valuable, he...erases you."

And then I knew what happened. I was making him—the Chameleon—a lot of easy money. Van must've become a big distributor for him once I was supplying cheap and high-quality goods. When I up and left, Van became less valuable and—

"You ran away right after I did," I said.

He nodded. "He would've killed me. With you gone, I was just an exposed liability. He doesn't like loose ends and if you're not profitable—he closes the branch and gets rid of the personnel. That's why he's been doing this for so long. He's good."

"How long has he been around?"

"Decades. He runs a lot of this city. Takes most stuff into his own hands. Things that you think would be beneath him, he personally takes care of it—gets some sort of twisted pleasure out of it. Makes him incredibly careful and incredibly dangerous."

I sighed and found a seat next to Van in some moldy leaves. "I'm sorry."

"Me too," he said before we shared some silence.

"He wants me to sell the half million worth of fentanyl I have on my own in a week."

"Not possible. He's toying with you."

"I know. But do you have any distributors you can refer? I'm desperate to unload and get out of this thing."

He shook his head. "Even if you sold all that, he'd just ask you to do it again—maybe even double it. He's never going to stop—he loves watching people squirm and squeal under his heel. I think you're more of a hobby to him at this point. Get out of state. Take your family and never come back."

"What about the DEA?"

"He's smarter than them. Smarter than you. You should leave, ASAP."

"What about you? You don't think he'd come looking for you in here?"

"Oh. I'm sure he will. For all I know, you just lead him directly to me."

I looked at him, both confused and terrified. "I swear no one followed me."

"His people are very good. They'll come sniffing around here soon—find out why you came here. They'll find me here." He gestured to the dead leaves scattered at his feet.

I shifted uneasily. How long had he been in business with the Chameleon? What kind of manipulation had that monster held over this...kid? And he looked more like a kid than ever, sitting cross-legged, gangly arms with disheveled hair. "Then get out of here. Come with me—we can figure something out.

Maybe we can plan something to trap him—set up a sting with the DEA…? Can you tell me anything about him? His name—other contacts?"

He laughed, and with an edge of hysteria in his voice said, "He's going to kill me, Dr. Rosen. I know he will—it's the consequence of my domino line." He looked off through the downtown buildings, a sliver of sunset catching his eye through the city.

"What?"

"I chose which domino to knock down, but I couldn't see how they would fall. I didn't know that this was all unavoidable after I knocked it down—after I got into this terrible game."

"But you don't need to just sit here..."

His vacant stare remained unbroken.

"Van, I'm...sorry."

"Don't need to apologize. I'm the one who goaded you into this whole thing. I was getting desperate for a new supplier."

"You can at least run. Get out of town."

He craned his neck, looking up at the clouds. "That's not what's in my dominos, anymore."

"Come on—remember when you told me that I can choose my own fate? You can do the same."

"I told you that because I wanted your supply."

"Still doesn't mean it's not true."

"The fate of the domino line is just that—fate. Neither good nor bad, it just *is*. Sometimes things will work out for you and sometimes they don't. The only constant is that there is a consequence."

I wasn't going to get through his hardened exterior of philosophy so I just asked, "Do you have...anything for protection?"

He shook his head. “I shed all my possessions. Just walking the earth now.”

“Here,” I said, handing my gun wrapped in a napkin. “Take it.”

“Not for me. No more.”

“Just take it!” I said, “even if you go throw it in the Sound right after. I want you to have it.”

He looked around and reluctantly took the gun.

“When the last domino falls on you, use it.”

He put the gun in his jacket—probably just to get rid of me. “You should go.”

I walked away without another word but then turned back. “Hey, Van?”

“Yeah?”

“Can you see my...aura?”

He squinted at me, confusion flooded his face. But then he nodded.

“And?”

“Pure gold.”

“What does that mean?”

“I guess someone still cares about you.”

I WANTED TO BE SMARTER.

And I wanted to be in a movie.

There’s always that rock-bottom moment that happens in the story—where everything is bad and then things get much worse. It’s when the viewer can’t possibly conceive a way out of the protagonist’s predicament. That’s where I was. And I wanted a writer pulling the strings behind me, feeding some brilliant plot twist into my subconscious that would solve all my problems in one elegant solution. Certainly there was some way to outsmart the Chameleon, but according to the script, I would need to sacrifice something that the Chameleon wouldn't expect. And that is how I would trick him: make his plans obsolete as I pulled a paradigm shift of what he believed my priorities to be.

This is why I wanted to be smarter. To outthink him. I wanted to throw the chess board in the air rather than keep moving pieces—always one step behind. But I wasn't that smart, and my life wasn't a movie—

Maybe a psychological thriller.

"Dad, " Regina said, waking me from my horrific reverie.

"What's up?" I said, stroking her hair.

"Can my new friend come over for a sleepover?"

"You've got a new friend on the block?"

She eagerly nodded, pigtails flailing behind her head. I hadn't seen her that excited in over a year. "Her name's Lacey."

"Sure, you can have her over."

"Thank you!" she said in a hurried whisper. She ran off like an excited little elf.

It killed me.

Her innocence. My guilt. My life had become some demented yin and yang of all my awful acts wrapped closely along the three most undeserving human beings in the world. I'd thought that Regina and Kris would be so much worse off without a father in their lives. But when it was *this* father sitting in the living room with them—they would flourish without my influence. I couldn't do it to them anymore. Every moment I spent with them was a crime.

Without realizing it, I was already too far down the hole. The moment I brought that first bag to Van—I'd fully stepped into a new, clandestine life with multiple interested and dangerous parties.

It was then that I knocked over the first domino.

"YOU NEED TO LEAVE."

Zella was distracted on her phone. "What?"

"You and the girls. You need to leave."

She covered the phone. "*Leave?*"

I nodded.

"Let me call you back," she said into the phone and hung up. "What are you talking about?"

"Pack your things, take the girls, and get out of town."

Her face went white. "Why are you saying these things?"

"I've...made some mistakes. Big mistakes. You can't be around me anymore."

"That's...okay. We can work through them."

I laughed.

"Don't laugh," she said.

"When will it ever be too much for you?"

"*What*?"

"At what point do you realize that I'm not worth it?"

"You—"

"I'm not who you think I am."

"That's—"

"Don't you have a shred of self-respect? Can't you see when a person in your life is nothing but poison?"

"Jude," she said through sudden sobs, "don't."

I held back tears. "You need to leave."

"Whatever it is, we can work through it."

I wanted to tell her everything at that moment—if only to convince her that our daughter's lives were in serious danger.

But I was scared. I was scared of going to jail—scared of never seeing my children again for the rest of my life.

She saw the wheels turning in my mind and asked, "Tell me. Whatever you did, you can always come back from it."

I hesitated. She would never understand.

"Was it Farrah?" she asked.

"Farrah?"

"Before she got sick?"

I was confused at what she was getting at and then understood. I nodded. "Yes."

"You were...with her all along?"

I nodded again. It wasn't true but it was the perfect excuse to get her and the girls out of the house. In order to get her as far away as possible, I needed her very, very angry at me. "I'll give you some money. I want you to take the girls out of state. Don't tell me where you're going. Pack light—put everything into the car with the garage door closed. Don't tell anyone—not your work or your mom. And leave."

"Why are you saying these things?"

"I…"

"What else is going on?"

"I...can't...tell you."

She stood, her eyes loving and open—

And then she gave me the hardest slap across my face I've ever experienced in my life. I fell to the ground, my head spinning.

I think I passed out a little.

"That's for lying about whatever it is you think I'm too stupid to hear."

"I don't deserve you," I told her, tasting blood in my mouth. "Never did."

"You don't deserve me because you don't deserve yourself."

I couldn't argue with that.

"WHY AREN'T YOU COMING?" Regina asked.

I lied to her, explained that it would only be for a little while—that I'd see her again in a week. She didn't say anything back—no bratty retort. I stood on the porch as she slung a bright pink backpack over her shoulder and disappeared around the corner to the garage. I wondered if I'd ever be able to explain to her why I was the way I was.

I'd left soon after, but pulled my car just a block away to watch our house. After another hour, I saw the garage door open and Zella's car back out. I saw our girls in the back seat and allowed myself a moment of relief. They were leaving. I followed them to the gas station. Zella got out and pumped gas—her face stoic, brave. I didn't wonder if she was relieved—I knew it. I'd finally given her the classic excuse to ditch her loser husband—infidelity. No one could blame her, not even herself.

I kept my eyes on the gas station and all the surrounding streets. There were no parked cars—no one keeping watch. I followed them to the freeway onramp, assuring myself there weren't any tails. As Zella pulled onto the ramp, I pulled over and watched the car disappear onto the freeway, the sun dwindling on the horizon.

My girls were gone.

I WOKE up the next morning to an empty house, my stomach on fire. A stabbing pain pulsated just below my sternum. After vomiting in the toilet, I crunched on some Tums and put on some sweats and a T-shirt. I went to the garage and pulled out the bags of fentanyl that I was supposed to sell for half a million dollars in two days or else be murdered.

After opening the passenger door of my car, I placed them on the seat in plain sight. I pulled out of the garage and got on the freeway. The sky was gray with a slight wreath of pink at the edge of the horizon where the sun was rising. Rain droplets splashed on the windshield with the cadence of a metronome—some sort of countdown, I supposed.

I pulled off downtown. After sitting in morning rush hour for another thirty minutes, I parked in front of a gray building with black tint windows and an ever descriptive sign that read "Municipal Center". I would have no idea that it was the DEA offices for Washington State if I hadn't visited once before and been accused of murdering my best friend.

I glanced over at the liters of fentanyl sitting on the passenger seat. I don't remember thinking much then—my movements and thoughts becoming robotic. I gathered the fentanyl into a plastic grocery bag and got out. After dutifully paying the parking meter, I walked up the long steps to the building.

I stood for a moment, listening to the wind. I felt relieved for the first time in a while. The girls were safe and I wouldn't have to have a secret life anymore. For the first time ever, justice was suddenly beautiful. I felt the veil of misery begin to lift from me. I was going to be free from myself—free from the exponentially poor decisions of Doctor Jude Rosen.

And then my phone rang.

Restricted number.

"...hello?" I said.

"813 Sunburst Terrace," the voice said, "don't be stupid." And then the line went dead.

I knew that address—but I didn't know how. I repeated it over and over again, but couldn't remember. I went to my contacts in my phone and typed in the address into the search bar—there was one hit.

Zella's sister in Oregon.

That's where they went.

And the Chameleon knew—he was watching me at that exact moment.

If I walked through the doors, my girls were dead.

I DIDN'T GET to Farrah's cabin till late that night.

After the phone call, I shrank from the DEA office and drove to the beach. I watched the waves of the Sound lap on the pebble beach for several hours. After that phone call, there was no more scheming—no more options.

I saw her cabin in my headlights, through the limbs of forest trees. I had no idea if it had been sold or still sat there vacant. I got to the front door and tried my key in the lock—

It still worked.

"Hello?" I said to the darkness. "Hello?"

No answer. No life within.

The place smelled of dust and cleaning supplies. I turned on the lights. Everything was exactly the same—Farrah's couches and chairs in the same position. Why hadn't anything been moved? Wasn't the cabin sold already? I realized I should've been around after her death, helped her family with the affairs but I wasn't even sure if they'd flown in—they certainly weren't at her funeral. I wondered what had happened to her little dog as I climbed the narrow staircase to the loft.

Her bed was still there.

I laid in it.

"Wish you were here," I said to the room. If only she could've been there to guide me—tell me how stupid I was and give me the solutions she always had for me. While it was true I never was technically unfaithful to Zella, I could never fully let go of Farrah. Maybe if she hadn't gotten sick—hadn't cooped herself up in a cabin to die—I would've finally cut the umbilical cord and given Zella all the love she deserved.

I let myself cry there for a good moment. I'd never felt more of a monster than sobbing about the tragedy of my life in the very spot where I had let her die—caused her death.

I stumbled back down the steps and sat on the couch. I wiped the tears away and then brought the plastic bag into my lap. I removed a half liter bag of fentanyl and found a notch on the overhanging lamp on which to hang it.

The entire day I knew what I was going to do. I was surprised I even made it up the steps of the DEA. I'd thought for a moment I could get immunity—get away with jail time for offering information about the Chameleon. But I didn't know a damn thing about him.

I'd always been a coward. I knew what the newspapers would say—knew the disgrace and harm that would come to my girls for the rest of their lives. But there was nothing else for me.

So I wrapped a tourniquet around my arm.

I placed an IV in my hand.

I attached the fentanyl bag to the IV.

The Chameleon would stop—leave the girls alone forever. It was a happy coincidence that I didn't really want to live anymore. I remembered Van's stupid words about the line of dominos. I couldn't have known—knocking over that first domino when I brought Van opiates—I couldn't have known that they would fall this way.

I kept the roller clamp in my hand—the switch to infuse the fentanyl. My thumb was over the clamp, keeping the infusion from flowing. Once I switched the clamp wide open, I would get the entire bag—twenty five grams of fentanyl—into my body in three to four minutes.

I heard words blooming in my mind—the mantra I'd say to myself:

There is no day without night.

There is no health without disease.

There is no life without a killer.

There is no joy without Jude.

It was time to meet my work partner—after all those years pumping on people's chests—we would see there was no difference between me and Death. Perhaps I could address Him as my friend. And maybe—

Maybe Farrah would be there.

THE WORLD WAS ABOUT to be a much, much better place without Doctor Jude Rosen.

CHAPTER NINETEEN

And then a really annoying thing happened.

I noticed an envelope sitting on the coffee table. It was unusual as the rest of the cabin was immaculately clean. I ignored it for a moment but then squinted at the envelope and saw: *For Dr. Jude Rosen*, scrawled in pen with a small Post-it and business card attached.

It could only be more bad news.

I looked up at the shimmering bag of fentanyl above my head, felt the clamp in my hand, and reluctantly let go. I picked up the envelope. The Post-It read:

Dr. Rosen,

I've been trying to get in contact with you at your home and hospital but without success. This letter was found next to Miss Abdi's body. Hoping it finds you here. Please call me as soon as you get this message.

Best, Judy Cliver, Esq.

Who?

I ripped open the envelope and unfolded the letter. It was Farrah's handwriting—wild loops and uncontrolled tails all over the place:

Jude,

Stop it.

Stop blaming yourself. This wasn't your fault. Death was coming for me. I needed to go on my own terms. This was my decision.

We were a miserable pair. Couldn't be together, couldn't be apart. If one of us was up, the other was down. I'm happy though, knowing that at least one of us has a halfway normal life. Tell Zella I love her. Tell your girls Aunt Farrah loves them always.

With all the doom and gloom we brought ourselves, try not passing it along to your girls. Be better for them, not for me.

I love you forever,

Farrah

I remembered when I saw her body in that bed—I'd flung the bedsheets away before collapsing on the floor. The suicide note must've gone tumbling somewhere. I let the letter drop to the floor. How did she do it? To lecture me—even from the grave? I was almost out.

Damn her.

I removed the fentanyl from my IV. It was not as if anything had changed. But, as usual, Farrah reminded of the terrible decision I was about to make. It only solved problems for Jude Rosen, but left the catastrophe he created behind for the rest of the world to deal with.

"Fine," I said to the silence, "fine."

MY PHONE RANG about an hour later.

It was Lazlo reminding me that I was late for my night shift. I wanted to tell him that—ha ha—he was lucky he caught me before I offed myself. Apparently the rest of the world hadn't yet caught up to what I was and I was still gainfully employed as an anesthesiologist.

So I drove to work. Because—

I couldn't think of anything better to do.

I had one day to sell all the fentanyl. Which was going to be difficult given that I'd dumped it all out in the bushes outside Farrah's cabin. As I pulled away, initially planning on booking it to Oregon where Zella and the kids were, I saw a car tailing me. They may as well have been driving a Zamboni—they weren't trying to hide from me anymore. The Chameleon wanted me to know he was watching everything I did. I tried calling Zella several times—telling her to get out of her sister's house but she didn't want to answer a call from her unfaithful husband at that moment.

So going to work seemed like the most benign choice. If anything, it would buy me time. The Chameleon would think I was trying to get more supply to sell, might make him give me an extension. And who knew—maybe the guy would just take the bulk fentanyl even if I couldn't sell it. Maybe he was actually just a really nice guy.

I'd lost the tail sometime in route—didn't see anyone behind me as I pulled into the parking garage. As I got out, I half expected the Chameleon to spring out any moment from the shadows, reminding me that I was going to die soon, etcetera, etcetera. But the garage was still as I walked in—the blast of air conditioning flowing through my hair. The sterile air cleared my mind. I was at work—the only place in my life I'd ever felt in control. I touched Farrah's memorial plaque as I passed by the OR front desk and made my way to the locker room, feeling strangely euphoric.

I found Lazlo at the front desk. "Sorry I'm late."

"Please don't make a habit of it. I had to cover for you."

I put my hand on his shoulder, realizing it might be the last time I'd see him or even step foot in the hospital. "I'm sorry, Dr. Lazlo."

He looked at my hand, confused.

"I'm sorry about everything. Sorry about the lawsuit—sorry for being an asshole." It must've been what it feels like to be on death row. All the petty nonsense of your life just melts away.

"That's...quite all right. Mind if I go home now?"

"Sure, boss."

As night came, the ORs started to close out their cases so I sent other providers and residents home for the night, keeping a few behind in case of an emergency trauma case. Soon, all the ORs were empty.

As I laid down in the call-room, the darkness enveloped me. Nothing had changed—I was in the exact same position. I was stalling. I pulled a business card out of my wallet—from the DEA agent who brought me in. It was late but he probably wouldn't mind that I was calling to confess to some very serious crimes that would probably land him some sort of promotion. Maybe he could get the police to Zella and the kids before the Chameleon could find out.

I took a deep breath—

And then a Trauma Code went off.

I BOLTED out the call room and flew down the stairs to the ER. I found the typical crowded resuscitation bay: nurses, surgeons, ER docs—everyone shouting and most people just getting in the way. An EMS was babbling out some sort of report—gunshot wound victims, one found dead at the scene, the other intubated and brought to the hospital by ambulance.

I elbowed my way to the bed and discovered a thin male with three bullet holes in his abdomen, one in his right chest. Each hole oozed with dark blood as the man coughed against the tube in his throat, flailing with every breath. As nurses started poking him up and down his arms, I saw his blood pressure start dipping: 90/50...80/45...70/30...

"Blood!" the ER doc yelled. "Give me four packed red and four plasma. Now!"

I got to the head of the bed and inspected the breathing tube. It was well secured with a decent carbon dioxide reading, meaning the EMS didn't accidentally stick it in the esophagus thinking they were ventilating the lungs. There was a good amount of blood coming out of the breathing tube—the bullet had gone through lung and perhaps some of the larger cardiac vessels. I inspected the patient's scalp, feeling for any missed shots to the head, but he looked clean. We pumped in the blood products but his blood pressure went down as his heart rate went up.

He was bleeding internally—fast.

Unzipping his belly and getting elbow deep would probably be the quickest fix for him. I looked at the surgeon. "Think we need to go to the OR?"

She shrugged. "Probably. I don't think we're plugging those holes with all that blood product."

"Let's go!" I yelled, unlocking the wheels of the gurney. I pushed through the crowd and took over ventilating—more blood came up through the tube. A lot more. "Think he may need a sternotomy, too," I yelled at the surgeon. "He's got a lot of blood coming from the lungs."

"We'll see."

We crashed him to the OR. I hooked him up to the anesthesia machine and slammed in some midazolam and fentanyl—I didn't want him remembering much more of the awful surgical things that were about to happen to his body. I bled in a trickle of anesthetic gas, isoflurane, just enough to give some sedation but not too much to tank his blood pressure. I then flushed in rocuronium—a potent paralytic so his body wouldn't move.

"Go!" I said.

The surgeon plunged a scalpel below the sternum and pulled down like she was starting a lawn mower. Within ten seconds, she had the bowel out, going over every inch with her fingers—searching...searching…searching. "Here," she said, "suture." As she tied off one bleeder, she found another and started working on the next. Meanwhile, his blood pressure was a dumpster fire.

"I don't think you're finding it," I yelled, "we're still losing blood somewhere. I'm going to do a central line." I called for an ultrasound machine, splashed some iodine on his neck, wrenched his head to the side and put a needle down his jugular. Once I knew I was clear of the carotid, I threaded a wire down and then railroaded a big ass catheter down to his heart. I called for a rapid transfuser and started pumping in blood products at light speed. I looked at his blood pressure—

70/30.

"You're not finding it!" I yelled. I started vasoconstrictors: first phenylephrine, norepinephrine, then vasopressin...then epinephrine. I looked back at the blood pressure—

60/20.

"He's going to arrest!" I yelled and then called for pads in case we needed to shock him. "I've got him on four pressors and giving round the clock blood. I don't think he's bleeding in his belly anymore—it's coming from somewhere else."

"Fuck!" the surgeon said. "Someone hand me a scalpel." A scrub nurse slapped one in her hand. She sliced the skin over the heart. "Saw!" The whir of a bone saw barked into life behind her. She grabbed it, flipping the switch on and brought it down to the patient's sternum. Flecks of bone and tissue aerosolized into the air as she cleaved the man's chest in two. "Rib spreader!" A saw-toothed extension with two metal prongs was brought to the man's chest. She fit the prongs snug within the bone groove and then twisted the lever—centimeter by centimeter. There was silence as she twisted until—

Crack.

His ribcage finally opened up like a stubborn clam.

And then a geyser of blood erupted from his chest. She plunged her hand into the cavern while the room went silent. "Ascending aorta," she said, "there's a hole."

"Bypass!" I yelled, "We need cardiopulmonary bypass!"

While I pumped in blood, a perfusionist rushed in with

what can only be described as a meth lab on wheels—pumps, tubing, meters and gauges all tacked together in line and assembled to completely drain the blood from someone's body, oxygenate it and then pump it back it. The only way to get control of a hole near the heart—is to stop the heart. That way the surgeon can actually see just what in the hell is going on enough to repair the damage.

So we primed the bypass machine, gave two ends to the surgeon and she jammed them in. We held a collective breath as the purple blood drained from his right atria, dumped into the bypass machine and then came back out cherry red—ready to flood back into the body.

"Go!" I told her.

As she plunged back into the chest, I kept filling him up with blood. I looked at the floor—it was covered with about one hundred spent bags of red blood cells, plasma, platelets and cryoprecipitate. He was still on max vasoconstrictors. The only other thing I could do to help his bleeding was make sure he was warm—cold patients can't clot. So I looked at the monitor to see his body temperature but realized I hadn't yet placed a temperature probe. I grabbed a probe from my cart and stepped up to the patient's head. I started to thread the temperature probe down the man's nose and finally noticed his face and then—

I fell over, a thunder clap of shock striking every nerve in my entire body.

It was...him.

It was *him.*

The Chameleon was on my table.

MOST OF THE TIME, the system of creating doctors works.

99.9% of the time, you can trust your anesthesiologist to monitor your sedated and paralyzed body.

But there's always that 0.1%.

That one vulnerable window where your anesthesiologist just isn't having a good day. And what if—

What if *you're* the reason he's not having a good day?

We're the doctors behind the curtain, behind the surgeons—

Behind the shadows.

We can do anything we want.

2ccs.

That's all it would take.

I could give him just 2ccs of any number of drugs and it would kill him almost instantly. Potassium chloride, concentrated epinephrine, vasopressin or phenylephrine. I could simply give him an overdose out of an entire drawer of drugs I had at my immediate disposal: metoprolol, labetalol, propofol, amiodarone, calcium chloride, neostigmine, atropine, hydralazine or lidocaine. I could just crank up the anesthetic gas and crash his blood pressure. Most of the drugs have short half-lives so even if there was an autopsy with a drug intoxication panel—nothing unusual would show up.

I could just turn the oxygen off—stop ventilating his lungs—and watch him suffocate.

I also could just...do nothing—

Step away.

The man was bleeding out of his aorta. He was needing continuous blood transfusions just to stay alive. I could just...stop. Doing. Anything.

Watch him crash and burn.

The answer to all my problems—the only definitive way to dig myself out of the hole I dug—was laying right in front of me as helpless as a person can be.

I'D ALREADY SAVED SO many murderers in the OR—wouldn't letting this one go kind of...even things out?

I'm not sure how my heart weighed in against a feather but I was certain I needed a different scale—my heart may have weighed a thousand pounds but there *had* to be more than one feather on the other end of the scale. I'd saved men who murdered children—gangsters and rapists. I'd also saved grandmothers, premature babies and competitive athletes. But I'd failed to save the patient with liver cirrhosis who bled out of every orifice. I'd failed to save the weekend warriors—the father of six who collapsed while playing football on Thanksgiving. I'd watched a teenage boy close his eyes for the last time in front of me—

I never thought there was anything special about it. It was just a Big Sneeze.

And then when you mix in all my recent drug dealings, marital manipulation, bad-dad complex and supplying a lethal dose of opiates to my best friend—

Where, exactly, was I going to weigh in?

I traced the dots of my recent life:

History of drug diversion, sick best friend who needs drugs, divert drugs, get into a multi-million dollar lawsuit leading to bankruptcy, selling drugs, drug lord wants to kill me and my family—drug lord shows up on my OR table...

It all made sense like some slippery-slope, Shakespearean tragedy of the anti-hero. Maybe becoming a killer is not a spontaneous act—but a gradual grooming of who you are. Life whittles you down from a blunt tree branch into a pointy-tip with the only remaining function of taking life when needed. Or maybe I was always a killer—a dormant beast kept at bay by suburbia life. Take those things away, and what was left? Or had my circumstances created me? Would the same thing have happened to anyone in my place?

I don't ask stupid questions anymore.

"DR. ROSEN, HE NEEDS BLOOD!" the surgeon yelled at me.

I snapped out of the shock and looked down at the Chameleon's face—pallid, cold and rigid. Not unlike when he was awake. I didn't know what cosmic event brought him to me but I had a choice to make and I had to make it fast. This man—my patient—was going to kill me if I didn't kill him. He wasn't just going to kill me—

He was going to kill my girls.

"He's oozing at the cannulation site!" she yelled, "give him something—anything!"

"Got it!" I moved into action and hung up another two bags of blood with some plasma. "I'll give him some Amicar," I said and went to my anesthesia cart. Instead of picking up the medication that could help his blood clot, I picked up a vial of nicardipine—a potent antihypertensive. It was a concentrated vial, intended to be diluted into a large bag of saline. Instead of diluting, I drew up the concentrated medication into a syringe and turned to the patient—to the Chameleon. With the man's blood pressure tanking, the last thing he needed was a ultra-high dose of a medication that was going to drop it further.

I held the syringe to his IV port.

Just a little squirt—and it would be over.

I had always been a partner with Death unto an end. There

is no life without a killer and there is no death without a healer. When death becomes so routine, the boundaries between who is doing the good and who is doing evil don't just blur—the distinction is ablated. Sometimes people lived and sometimes they died—

But mostly they died.

CHAPTER TWENTY

"Do you know where you are?"

He opened his eyes, squinting at the ceiling. "Muh?"

"Do you know what city you're in?"

He brought his face to mine, his eyes still adjusting. "Seattle," he said before coughing up phlegm.

"We were able to get the breathing tube out just now."

"Thank you. What...what happened?"

"You're in the hospital. In the ICU."

"How?"

"Yes. You're *very* lucky to be alive."

"But...what happened?"

"You went looking for Van. And you found him."

He perked up, craned his neck, and gazed at me—realization blooming.

"He was right about his line of dominos—that he couldn't avoid it—couldn't avoid you. Did he see *my* dominos, though? Me and you, across from each other, talking about what happens next?"

The man clenched his fists and tried sitting up but gasped from pain. He clutched his chest.

"Had to crack your chest open—probably a little painful. Took hours to fix you up."

He craned his neck, looking for anyone else.

"No, no. It's just me and you right now. Focus up. I didn't really believe his palm-reading mystic bullshit myself but I got to say—there's something weird about me and you meeting up this way, isn't there? Maybe there is some sort of saving grace for someone like me despite all the incredibly stupid things I've done. You laying in that gurney right now is proof enough for me. Someone out there is still looking out for me but I don't think it's for my benefit—I'm not that great."

His gaze turned cold, his eyes fixed on mine.

"You did kill Van, by the way, but not before he left four bullets in you—one in your aorta. Don't worry. I was your anesthesiologist. I kept you safe...the entire time."

"What did you do to me?" he hissed.

"Ask me why you're alive right now." Beneath his eyesight, I was holding a syringe in my hand, the end of which was attached to his IV tubing.

"You have no idea what I'm going to do to you."

"Ask me why you're alive right now," I repeated.

"You think because I'm in this bed that you're *safe*? This changes nothing."

"I see. You think we're still out there," I said, waving to the window, "on the streets—your world. No. You're in here—in my world. In here...I'm always in control."

He snorted. "Fine. I'll give you a small extension on the deadline. Get me a phone. I'll tell my people."

"Hmm. I can see you still don't understand. Let me...*help you*." I pushed down on the plunger of the syringe, shooting the liquid into his IV. I then flipped on the sound of his oxygen saturation. It had the high beep of someone with one hundred percent oxygen in their blood. "In a few seconds, you're going to start feeling....strange."

"If you touch me, your family is—" His eyes became unfocused.

"I just gave you one hundred milligrams of a drug called rocuronium. It's a potent neuromuscular paralytic. It works in about twenty seconds and paralyzes every muscle in your body—including your diaphragm. You know...the one that helps you breathe? I usually give people a sedative before giving rocuronium as it has a tendency to make someone feel like they're in a coffin within their own body."

He gasped and tried to speak, but the drug had settled in. His expression petrified into one of horror as he became still—his body now a statue of flesh.

"That's better," I said. "Now to answer my earlier question: why are you alive right now? I keep asking myself that question. Not only were you lucky to survive that injury, but the man whose job it was to keep you alive for eight hours of surgery happened to be a man whose wife and children you threaten to have murdered. I had a million chances to blink you into oblivion without a soul questioning—would've solved all my problems."

His eyes were open but he didn't blink. His jaw slack.

"I don't think I kept you alive out of benevolence. I wholeheartedly want you dead."

His oxygen saturation started to dip down to the low nineties as he remained completely motionless.

"Because, I am, in fact...not a good person."

The room was still. No nurses—nobody around.

"Fortunately for you, I have actual good people in my life

—people that don't really know what I am."

His oxygen dropped to the mid-eighties.

"And I would actually like to someday undo the harm I've caused. Not sure if I have any chance of that happening, but I am sure if I murdered a helpless patient in cold blood—that there's no coming back from that. It's also not a good start in life for two little girls when their dad is a murderer."

His oxygen was in the mid-seventies—his lips blue.

"Are you uncomfortable?"

His oxygen dipped lower, his heart rate dropping. At that moment the man was wide awake, air hunger driving him mad, feeling every moment of suffocating.

"Here," I said, bringing an oxygen mask to his mouth. I gave him a few breaths till his oxygen came back to the nineties. I walked over to the computer and turned on the screen. "You know, you learn a lot from someone's medical chart, Mr. Novak. Mr. Patrik Novak at 831 Steeplechase Dr. A lot of valuable information for law enforcement." I glanced at him. His body still as motionless as a corpse. "I think I know everything I need to know about you. Just in case we have any more...problems. I also want you to remember how you feel right now—remember what I can do to you."

His oxygen started dipping again.

"Oh, I'm sorry. Let me take care of that for you." I brought out another syringe and attached it to his IV tubing. "This is suggamadex. It'll bind up that nasty paralytic and have you dancing right out of here." I pushed the drug.

In eight seconds, the Chameleon jerked awake, his limbs thrashing as he choked on the air. His chest heaved up and down as he tried to catch his breath. He glared at me with the rage of a man who hadn't been challenged in a very long time.

A child's voice rang out from behind me. "Daddy!"

I turned and saw two small children run into the room—a woman behind them holding an infant. The woman looked at the Chameleon and said, "He's awake!"

"Yes," I told them, "and he's doing great."

"Are you his doctor?" she asked.

"Yes. I was his anesthesiologist during the case. He was in critical condition when he came in but he pulled through. We were able to get the breathing tube out just a few moments ago. He's still a little short of breath." I looked at him and received a cold stare. "Are you his wife?"

"Yes. These are his kids. We were..." she fought back tears, "so worried about him."

"Well you shouldn't have anything to worry about now."

His little girl came up and tugged on my scrubs. "Doctor?"

"Yes?"

"Is my daddy going to be okay?"

I scooped up the little girl and bounced her in my arms. "Oh yes," I said, brushing her hair out of her eyes. "Isn't that right, Mr. Novak?" I asked, turning to the Chameleon.

He looked at me, still breathing heavy.

"We're not going to have any more problems. Are we, Mr. Novak?" I asked again.

He looked from me, to his wife and then to his little girl cradled in my arms.

"No," the Chameleon said. "No more problems."

I WALKED out of the hospital and looked over the harbor. The sky was clear with a layer of pink clouds crowding the horizon. I had felt so triumphant, belittling the man as I paralyzed his body. It should've felt as if all my problems had melted away. But standing there, taking in the beauty of dawn, it was as if I'd fallen asleep hungry and dreamt I had a feast only to wake again to starvation. A quiver of anxiety hummed within me—robbing what should've been my triumph. Knowing the Chameleon wasn't after me or my girls—did nothing. The only thing that would restore who I was—the person I'd become—was to get my girls back.

I KNOCKED on the door and waited.

Zella opened.

I fell into her arms. Her sweater dampened as I sobbed harder than I ever had. She held me until I ran out of breath and then stroked my hair.

"Are you ready?" she asked.

I beheld her—resplendent with understanding. I nodded. I was so afraid—afraid to say another word. A dread had grown within me as I drove to Oregon—some sort of deep suspicion about life and redemption.

"You're ready to tell me the truth?"

I nodded and dumped everything on her.

SHE PROMPTLY DIVORCED ME.

I had imagined coming home to my girls, taking them into my arms and whisking them to the park. I could put the last year out of my life forever—return everything back the way it was. But that wasn't going to happen. My suspicions about life were true: when lies replace truth, all that's left is rot. And I had rotted to the core.

Zella told the DEA everything.

I was arrested at my home, alone.

They brought me in, prepared to dazzle me with their

investigative wiles but I just dropped the whole story in their laps before they could get a word out. I didn't give any details about who the Chameleon actually was until they asked.

"Is immunity a thing or is that just in movies?" I asked them.

They looked at one another and both said, "We'll see."

I gave them every ounce of information I knew about Patrik Novak—not until they guaranteed me no jail time.

But they sent me to jail anyway.

Minimum security, two years, then house arrest. It was a better deal than anything I could've expected. Apparently bringing down Novak was kind of a big deal and they didn't care a whole lot about some loser anesthesiologist being a short term supplier as long as he lead to the arrest of the biggest drug kingpin in the city.

The time alone proved fruitful: I pondered, I prayed, I read—

And I wrote.

"YOU HAVE A VISITOR," a guard told me.

I wanted to skip down the hallway, thinking Zella had finally come to see and speak to me for the first time. But it wasn't her or my girls. Sitting opposite the glass partition I found an older woman with a slanted mouth painted in bright red lipstick.

"Hello?"

"Dr. Rosen," she said. "It's nice to finally meet you. You're a hard person to get a hold of. Don't you ever pick up your phone or check your mail?"

"I'm not a doctor anymore."

"Right," she said, "my apologies."

"What is this about?"

"My name is Judy Cliver. I was the estate lawyer for the late Farrah Abdi."

"Oh."

"Did you find the note I left for you in your cabin?"

"Yes. It saved my life."

She tilted her head, nonplussed.

"And don't you mean Farrah's cabin?"

"No, Mr. Rosen. I mean *your* cabin. I think we have a lot to talk about."

WHEN I WAS RELEASED from prison, I was the sole inheritor of Farrah's estate.

2.3 million dollars.

Plus a cabin.

If I had only picked up the damn phone.

I was soon out of jail and flush with cash. And like some twisted fairy tale ending, everything worked out for your boy, good old Jude Rosen.

Everything—

Except I was a miserable monster of a man.

AND THAT'S why I wrote this—I wanted you to understand me.

Sitting there, newly imprisoned, I was suddenly empathetic of all the mass murderers, serial bombers, and arsonists during their media courtroom appearances. I never felt some sort of sycophantic kinship with them. No, I just saw them with different eyes. They all say the same thing that I wanted to say:

You haven't heard my story.

And it's not as if they're innocent, but I thought maybe

there are small steps along the way that dragged them toward their acts. I doubt they all intended to be what they became. Perhaps there is value in listening to them—that they have something to teach us about ourselves. And so I wrote my story for you. I wanted you, above all people, to know why I did the things I did. I thought you'd learn from me.

I'd hoped to create context.

Context is a helpful thing. Sometimes it's important, other times it is crucial to understanding. Context turns villains into heroes. But most of the time, as I discovered, it's the opposite.

I know that, after reading my story, you might see why I did the things I did—you understand the small yet tragic failures in course correction. I'd hoped that it would provide the context to explain my actions. But, after writing this out and seeing it all unfold on these pages, context has not revealed what I wanted: that I was a person caught up in unusual circumstances which led to poor decisions. No, there's only one thing to learn from my story:

Context is for the wicked.

IT'S what your mom finally understood when I told her the truth. It's what Farrah never understood as she kept trying to help me throughout all those years—that I was only as good as the context surrounding me. I'd buffered in enough caring and motivated people that I'd never developed a real person inside. Once the buffer was gone, only the rot remained.

How do you apologize for being a bad person? Can I make it up for being gone for the rest of your childhood? Can I change the last memories you have of me—escaping in the middle of the night with your mom and baby sister while I stood on the porch? Can I take away the articles all over the internet about your psychopathic, doctor, drug kingpin of a father? Can I just say....that I'm *sorry*?

No.

With some mistakes, words will never be enough.

So here's the deal:

After dropping my story at your doorstep, I won't ever come back.

These words can be the last you'll ever hear from me if that's what you want. I'll just be the infamous bad dad who's rotting away somewhere. But, because I know you're far better than your dad ever was, you may want to find me. Because that's what good people do—they have hope. Even for all us sinners out there.

If you have that hope for me, you can find me. I'll be at Fair Haven rehab center for the homeless of Seattle. For some reason I got an extension on trying this thing out again—it's not every day that a murderous drug dealer falls into your lap. So, I donated half of Farrah's inheritance to the rehab center and spend most of my waking hours here now. It will take me the rest of my days to dig out of the hole of a person I created.

I think this will be a good start.

I think there are people here I can help.

And I think they can help me.

AND WHETHER YOU see me again or not, I'll always love you. Whatever you decide, Regina, there is a trust fund for you and Kris with the other half of Farrah's inheritance waiting for you when you're eighteen. Get an education if you want but more importantly, be kind and be willing to help others. There's nothing magic about it.

Be something better than your Doomy Gloomy Daddy.

AFTERWORD

Thank you for exploring the character of Jude Rosen with me. While I certainly pulled many concepts from my own life and fed them into the setting of the book, Jude himself is entirely fictional.

I'm grateful to the beta readers in my life who helped to make this book possible: Danny Allen, Craig Ebert, Ashley Pyne, Jessica Welker, Jackson Bladen, and of course my wife, Jillian Tovarek-Welker, who is the ever present sounding board off which I bounce thousands of ideas.

I'd also like to offer a special thank you to Linnerd and Dom Testa for their guidance to a budding author.

REVIEWS MATTER

As a HUGE reader of fiction myself, I carefully vet the books I read by reading reviews on Goodreads, Amazon and book blogs. No book goes anywhere without honest reviews.

If you enjoyed *Needle Work*, I ask that you take a moment to leave me a review. I read every review of everything I've written and I definitely respond to reader feedback. Thank you.

ALSO BY WICK WELKER

Medora

The Medora Wars

ABOUT THE AUTHOR

Wick Welker writes in multiple genres including medical, sci-fi, and fantasy. He is a medical doctor who practices critical care medicine and anesthesiology. While he claims Utah, Seattle and San Francisco, he currently calls Minnesota home with his wife and cat (who they worship).

Made in the USA
Coppell, TX
04 November 2026

11282154R00142